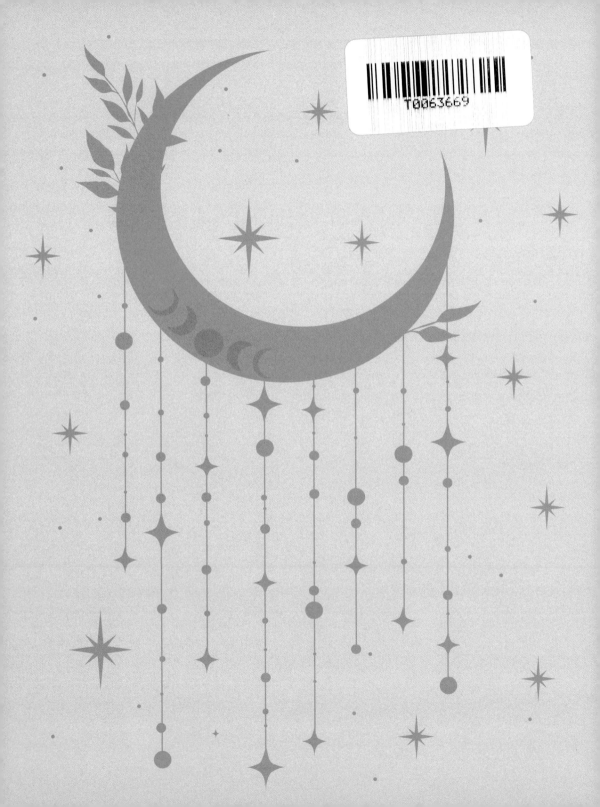

Glamour Magic

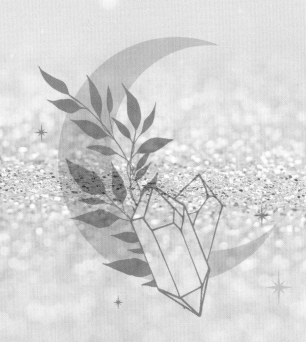

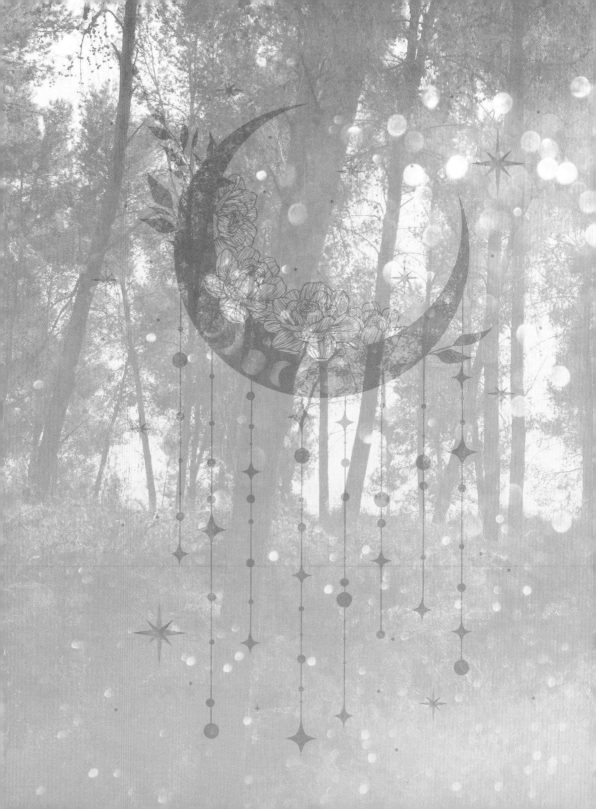

Glamour Magic

Enchantments to build confidence and beauty

Marie
Bruce

SIRIUS

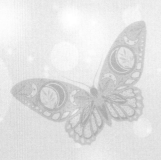
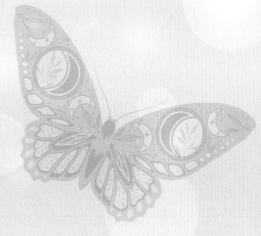

SIRIUS

This edition published in 2024 by Sirius Publishing, a division of
Arcturus Publishing Limited,
26/27 Bickels Yard, 151–153 Bermondsey Street,
London SE1 3HA

ISBN: 978-1-3988-3668-6
AD010565UK

All images courtesy of Shutterstock
Designer: Sally Bond

Printed in China

Contents

Mirror, Mirror, on the Wall

'*Mirror, mirror, on the wall*
Who is the fairest of them all?'

Have you ever felt more like the Wicked Queen than Snow White, or identified more closely with the old hag than the beautiful princess? If so, you may have refused party invitations, chickened out on dates and missed out on promotions at work because you just didn't feel good enough. Life isn't a fairy tale, but there is no reason why you can't learn to incorporate some fairy-tale glamour into your daily routine.

Glamour is a carefully crafted illusion and one that witches have used for centuries to cast an aura of power, mystery and seductiveness around themselves. It can make you stand out in a crowd, perform better in a job interview, have the confidence to go out on more dates, or seduce your partner when they least expect it. Glamour can help you to walk taller, stand straighter, speak out with authority on topics you are passionate about and generally move through life with more grace and wit than you had before. Glamour begins as an illusion that eventually becomes reality, and this means that anyone can achieve it. It doesn't depend on expensive lip fillers or Botox, nor must you spend hours in the gym. You can become glamorous regardless of your age, shape, size or gender, because glamour is for everyone. Everyone, that is, who wants to try it.

In this book you will learn about the power of glamour and glamour spells, how to cast magic with makeup, how to make beauty bias work to your advantage and how to cultivate an air of mystery and charisma.

Here you will learn how to charm with self-love rituals, climb the career ladder with the help of glamour spells and even how to become something of a femme fatale. So, grab your lipstick and dive with me into the world of beauty rituals and glamour-puss spells, because the world can be your oyster – you just need to learn how to captivate it. It's time to put your best face forward: your curtain call awaits!

Beautiful blessings,

Marie Bruce x

Chapter One

What Is Glamour Magic?

*What makes you different or weird -
that's your strength!'*

MERYL STREEP

Often when people think of witches, they call to mind storybook images of hook-nosed old hags, living in the woods and casting evil spells on any who cross their path. This is the stereotype that rears its ugly head every Halloween, yet as every Wiccan knows, it doesn't bear much resemblance to the truth. Real witches look much the same as anyone else: we have ordinary jobs, careers, hobbies and families. We live in ordinary homes. From the outside we seem just like everyone else. Yet there is something unusual about us, something that you might not be able to put your finger on. That something is *glamour*.

Glamour is our secret weapon. We wear it well, and it serves us even better! Glamour ensures that we get noticed in all the right ways and by all the right people. In a nutshell, glamour is the essence of a witch's power of attraction. It is how she views herself and her place in the world. It is how she presents and carries herself. It is her super-power and it can be yours too. I use the feminine pronoun because that is my personal experience, but there are lots of male and non-binary witches too, so use whichever pronoun you feel comfortable with. Glamour is for everyone.

WHY DO I NEED GLAMOUR MAGIC?

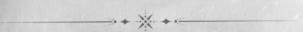

Good question! Glamour is a skill, which, when utilized correctly, can enhance your life and all your interactions. Whoever you are, whatever your current circumstances might be, glamour can help you to…

- Get the coveted job or a career other people can only dream of.
- Win the heart of your true love and chosen life partner.
- Captivate a room with ease.
- Master a board meeting.
- Win respect.
- Hold your own at a party or red-carpet event.
- Shine in an interview and get the job offer before you've even left the room.
- Speak your truth, expressing yourself clearly and eruditely.

- Have a string of suitors all vying for your attention.
- Receive small favours and little gifts from friends and strangers alike.
- Receive compliments and looks of appreciation, wherever you go.
- Create beauty in every aspect of your life.
- Live elegantly.

A glamorous witch leads a glamorous life. She brings beauty to her home, buying fresh flowers or tending her plants, lighting scented candles and choosing furnishings with care. If this doesn't sound like you, don't worry – it soon will be. Glamour is a lifelong journey and, like personal hygiene, it is something you should do every day to maintain the best effect.

WITCHES AND GLAMOUR

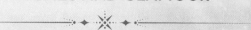

Witches have always been considered glamorous. In the time of the witch hunts, from the 14th to the 18th centuries, this could lead to a woman's downfall: she might find herself being accused of beguiling a man by witchcraft and be brutally murdered for it, by hanging or burning in a barrel. You only have to think of sorceresses such as Morgan le Fay in the Arthurian legends and Circe in Greek mythology to see that there has always been a very fine line between magic and glamour.

More recently in the 20th and 21st centuries, the media has glamorized witches in films and popular TV shows such as *Charmed* or *A Discovery of Witches*. The imagery used in these shows is a far cry from the warty green-skinned wicked witch of the past, and instead these modern fictional witches are shown as independent, feisty females who are quite capable of saving the world with a spell, and looking stunning at the same time.

So where does that leave us? How do modern witches find themselves and their glamour-power, firmly lodged as we are between these two extremes? In the past, glamour could get you killed; in the present, it is often seen as a beauty standard that is virtually impossible to achieve.

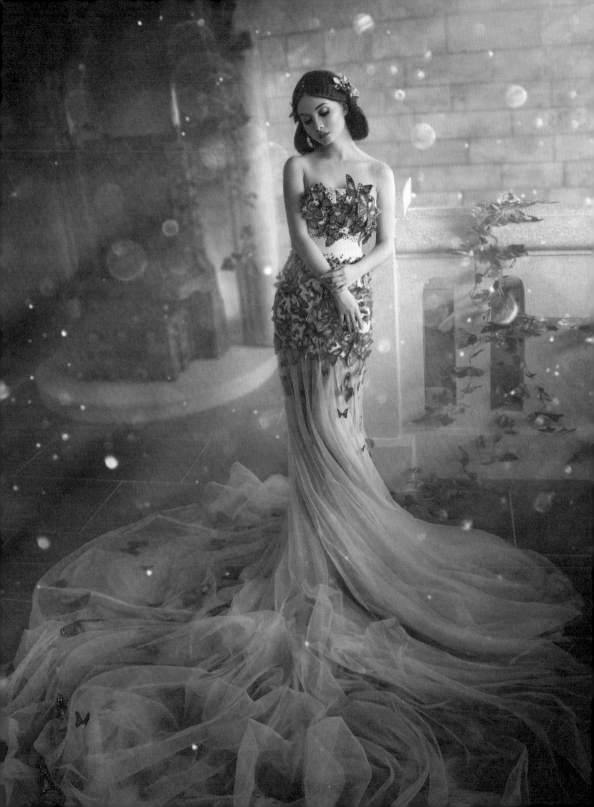

In the Cambridge Dictionary glamour is defined in the following way: 'The special, exciting and attractive quality of a person, place or activity.' According to this definition, glamour is about so much more than looks, natural beauty or personal appearance. It is a quality that has an emotional effect on the observer. It is something that draws people in and makes them want to stay a while. This is the kind of glamour we will be exploring in this book and, while personal appearance undoubtedly plays a part, it is not the be-all and end-all. You don't have to conform to certain beauty standards to be glamorous or to get the best out of your life using glamour spells.

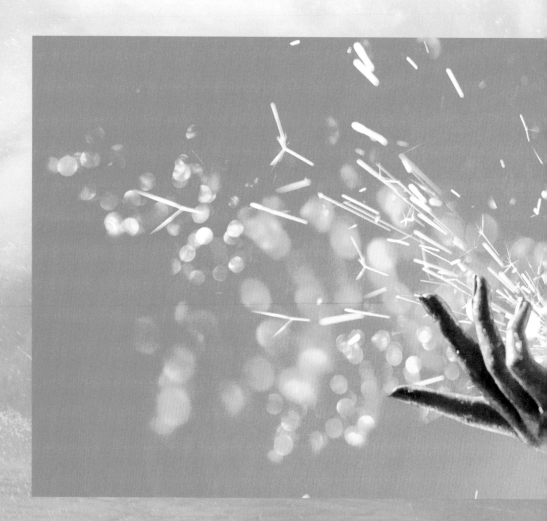

Glamour magic is about being the best version of yourself and using that personal power to live the best life you can. Now, when you really commit to *that* as a concept, you will soon see that all other external standards and expectations fall away quite naturally, because there is only one of you, so your standard of glamour will be unique to who you are and how you choose to express yourself. With this in mind, there should be no further need to lose sleep over the fact that you do not have, for example, the derrière of Kim Kardashian or Kylie Minogue. And, hopefully, you will discover that your own seat is quite peachy, nonetheless!

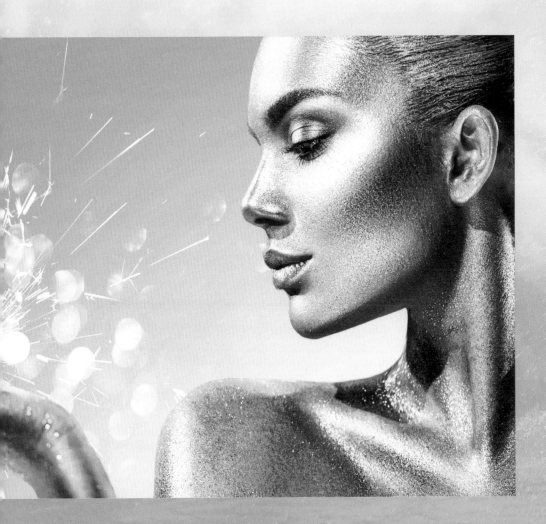

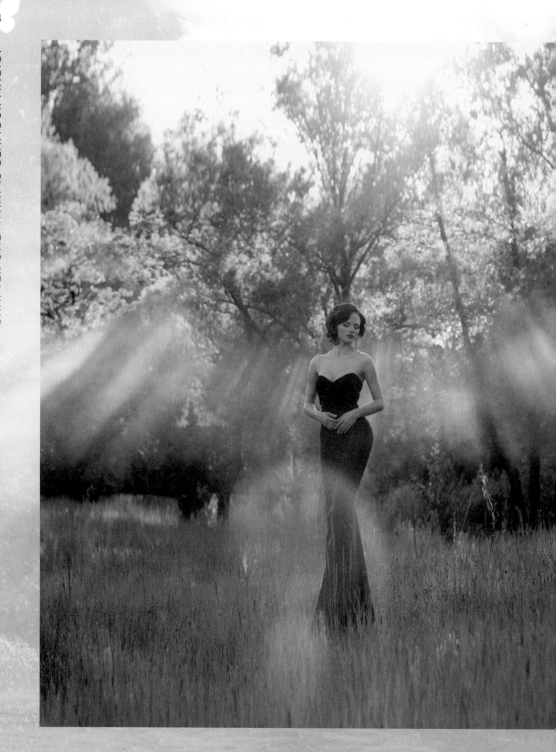

GLAMOUR IS FOR EVERYONE

Glamour isn't just for the rich and famous, the pop princesses and the Hollywood starlets. It's for everyone and while we are conditioned to believe that it is essentially a feminine trait, nothing could be further from the truth. In fact, a highly glamorous man can be a very powerful enticement indeed.

Glamour is a force to be reckoned with. It is a strong magnetic field that captivates your audience, reeling them into your orbit, compelling them to do nice things for you, just to make you smile. This isn't about manipulation. It is simply a natural consequence of you being your most charming and glamorous self, so enjoy the results!

WHERE DOES GLAMOUR COME FROM?

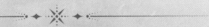

Glamour comes from within, from deep in your psyche and your soul. It isn't something that can be given to you by someone else. Glamour is a gift you give to yourself. It is a combination of confidence, elegance, grace, intelligence, education, wit, sensuality, humility and charm. All these things working together is what makes someone glamorous. Putting other people at ease is glamorous. Demonstrating good manners is glamorous. Etiquette is glamorous. And all these qualities are free for you to own and develop. It is down to you to take the time to nurture them, using the rituals, tips and tricks in this book.

CASTING GLAMOUR SPELLS

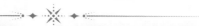

Glamour magic works in the same way as any other type of spell-casting. You must have a clear vision of your goal in mind as you cast and you should back up your spells in a real way. For instance, if you have had your eye on someone for a while and you want them to pay you more attention, you could cast a spell designed to get you noticed, then back up that spell by taking extra care over your appearance when you are likely to see the object of your desires – perhaps wearing something you would usually save for best.

In this way, not only are you giving yourself the best chance of getting that person to notice you, but you are also likely to attract the attention of other people too. When your love interest witnesses the attention you are receiving, they are more likely to be intrigued, because attracting attention from others will, in turn, make you more alluring to your target. Plus, it has the additional benefit of allowing you multiple chances to flirt and interact with other people too, so that you can perfect your charm offensive. It's a win-win result.

Glamour doesn't always require an audience, however. It can be just as effective when you are alone. There might be times, for instance, when you want to feel more glamorous specifically for your own amusement. Maybe you have new makeup or skincare products you want to try out and decide to dress for the occasion in a negligee, like a Hollywood starlet. Indulging in glamorous practices alone could be a positive way to soothe your ego after a romantic disappointment or to work on some self-love. Your glamour isn't only for the benefit of your significant other or fellow party guests, it is primarily for you. It is an aspect of your personality in which you should indulge on a regular basis. It is 'me time', rolled in sparkling diamond dust!

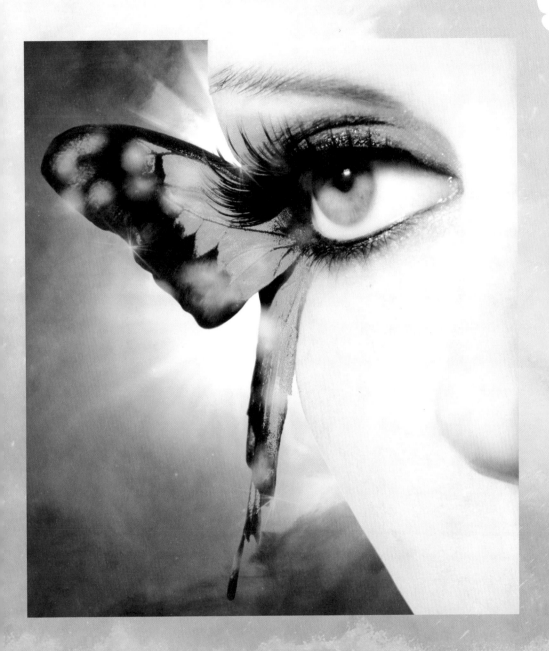

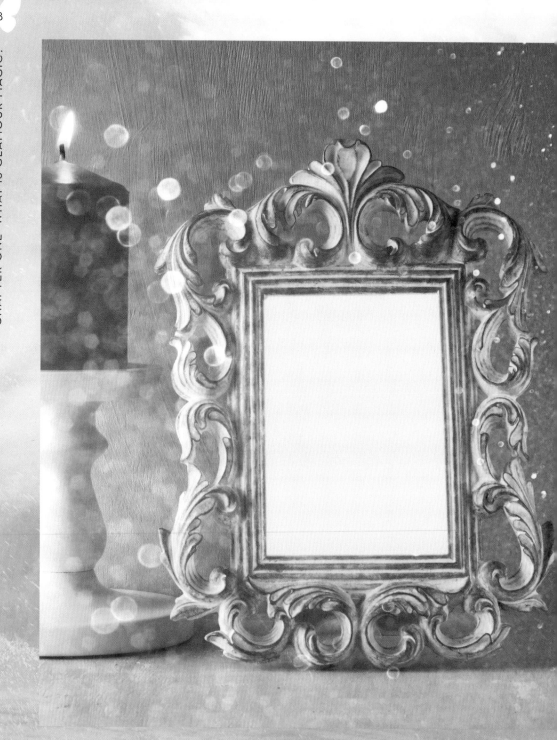

GLAMOURIES GALORE!

Glamourie is an old Scottish word that means enchantment or something or someone that is invested with magic. To 'have a glamourie on ye' means to have been touched by magic, either of your own conjuring, or someone else's. In this book you will find many *glamouries* for you to try out. These are simple spells and tips to help you to become more glamorous.

Glamourie: Mirror, Mirror

Some people dislike looking in the mirror. It brings up all kinds of emotions for them, from inadequacy to self-loathing, but it is something we all usually have to do when getting ready for the day, so instead of seeing the mirror as the enemy, turn it into a magical tool. Each morning as you stand in front of the mirror, look into your own eyes and say the following mantra as you get ready for the day ahead:

This is what a glamorous person looks like
I am what a glamorous person looks like
I am glamorous in all I do and say
I am glamorous every single day!

Chapter Two
Beauty Bias

'For beautiful eyes, look for the good in others...'

AUDREY HEPBURN

We all know that looking great on the outside can help us to feel good on the inside. This is because your personal presentation and self-image have a deep impact on your mental health. People who are depressed or bereaved often resort to wearing the same clothes over and over again because it is easier. They simply might not have the mental bandwidth available to put together nice outfits. Comfortable trousers and a baggy top can quickly become a go-to outfit every day – a uniform of misery.

I would argue, though, that it is when life is hard that you should take the extra time to make even more of an effort in your personal appearance, because it will help to lift your spirits, even if just by a small margin. This, in turn, can give you the boost you need to get through another day. The armed forces have a long history of teaching soldiers to scrub up and take care of their personal appearance because it is good for morale. So, when life gets difficult, think like a soldier and smarten up!

Appearance isn't everything, of course. Personality, a sense of humour, intelligence, honesty and so on are all very important in helping you to stand out from the crowd, but glamour simply wouldn't be glamorous if one's appearance wasn't taken into account. While today's beauty standards can be difficult to live up to, if not impossible, it will nonetheless serve you well if you strive to put your best face forward at all times. Not only will it boost your own confidence, but it will also have a positive impact on your life in general and the opportunities that come your way.

The simple fact is: beautiful people get ahead. This is because they naturally get more attention, more doors open for them and so their prospects are better. They receive greater opportunities and spontaneous favours from others. Life tends to run more smoothly for attractive people, meaning that success and prosperity can come to them more easily and, in turn, greater wealth and status make them even more attractive! In addition, attractive people tend to be forgiven for their transgressions more easily than those deemed to be less attractive, even if they step out of line – their beauty affords them a certain amount of protection.

All this is known as 'beauty bias' or 'pretty privilege'. It might not be a nice way to think about things, but it is the world we live in and the one we have to navigate. Beauty bias means that those considered to be conventionally attractive are more likely to get hired, promoted and invited on dates. It means that the prettiest in society will rarely be left stranded by the side of the road with a flat tyre, because someone will be drawn to their beauty enough to stop and help.

It isn't fair, but then life isn't always fair, is it? However, a touch of glamour can give you the tools you need to level up the playing field and you don't have to look like a supermodel or a film star to use beauty bias to your own advantage. You just need to ensure that you always look your best, especially when there is a big promotion at work up for grabs!

THE DOWNSIDE OF PRETTY PRIVILEGE

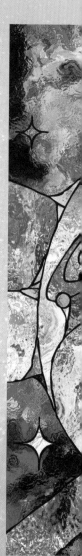

It might seem as if beautiful people have everything handed to them on a plate, but make no mistake, pretty privilege has its pitfalls too – the most obvious being unwanted, uninvited and unwelcome attention. This can range from a wolf-whistle in the street, or a flirty colleague lingering at your desk, to more serious crimes such as stalking or assault.

Of course, this issue is by no means something that only women experience; it can be challenging for any attractive person. In addition, the more glamorous and beautiful you are, the more likely it is that you will inevitably attract envy, jealousy and even, in extreme cases, hatred. Some people might try to compete with you, going out of their way to out-do you in all things. This type of 'keeping up with the Joneses' behaviour is a sign that people might be envious; that they want what you have and are using imitation to try and level up.

Others might become hostile as soon as you enter a room, or speak to their partner. They might indulge in obvious public displays of affection, or possessive body language, to demonstrate that their partner is off the market, when perhaps all you did was smile and say hello. This behaviour stems from jealousy, which is the fear of losing something – in this case, a partner.

It is important to remember that all these people are really doing is highlighting their own insecurity. Don't dignify their behaviour with a response, simply continue to be charming and polite, safe in the knowledge that your glamour has out-shone them and they are fully aware of it! How they deal with that is their own responsibility, not yours.

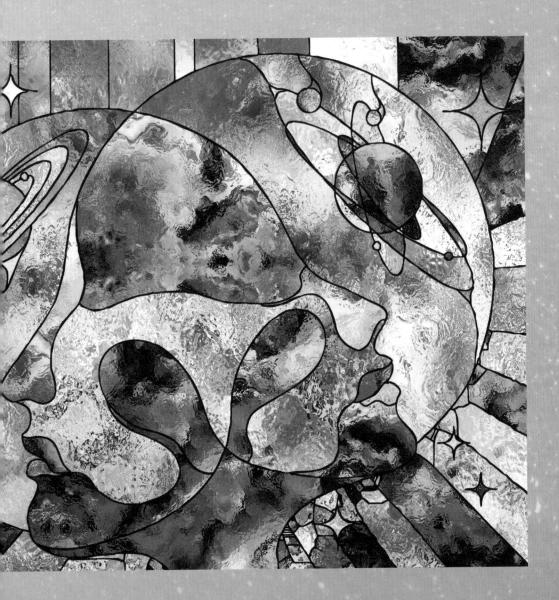

MAKING THE MOST OF BEAUTY BIAS

How do you ensure that beauty bias works in your favour? The most obvious answer is to make the best of yourself and downplay the bits you'd rather not draw attention to. We all have aspects of our appearance and personality we quite like and aspects we don't, so try to draw attention to your best bits. What matters most is not how attractive you are *per se*, but how well you can present yourself and show off your main attributes. That said, there are other things you can do to ensure that beauty bias isn't actively working against you.

MAKING BEAUTY BIAS WORK FOR YOU

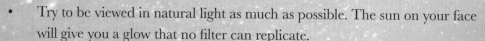

- Try to be viewed in natural light as much as possible. The sun on your face will give you a glow that no filter can replicate.
- Smile! This will open up your face and make you appear warmer and more welcoming.
- Look people in the eye, keeping your gaze soft and non-threatening.
- Keep your body language open, preferably with your palms on display to show that you have nothing to hide.
- Don't fidget. Try to move through the world with poise and elegance.
- Move gracefully and slow down. Rushed movements can make you clumsy.
- Take a moment to think before you speak, considering how you want to express yourself.
- If possible, try to put yourself in a place of beauty, allowing that beauty to enhance your own. A park, woodland, church or stunning building will all help to magnify your own beauty. Anne Boleyn allegedly used this trick by planning a meeting with King Henry VIII in a garden at Hever Castle, thus ensuring her beauty was enhanced by all the flowers around her.

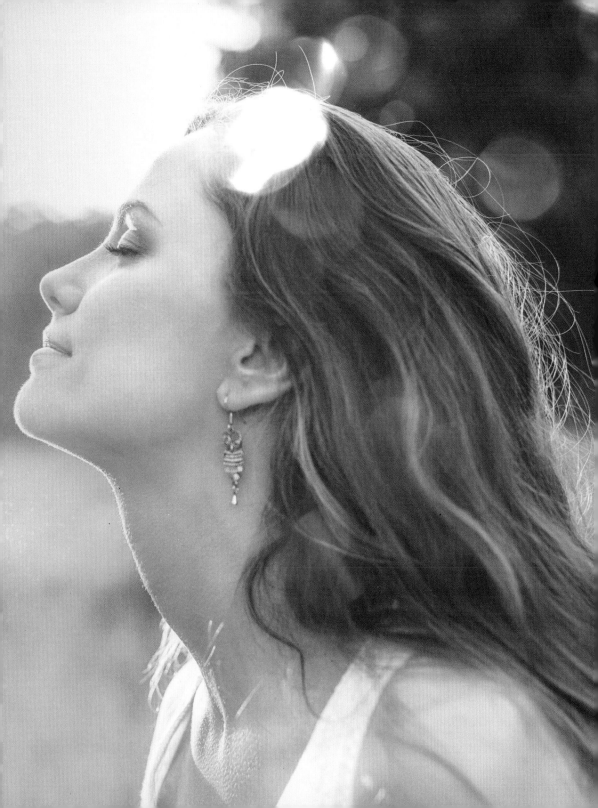

- If you can't place yourself in a landscaped garden, arrange things of beauty around you instead – flowers, crystals, flickering candles. Being surrounded by pretty things will make you seem more attractive.
- Remember your manners! Manners maketh man, or woman, considerably more attractive.
- Stand and sit tall, don't slouch but carry yourself well. No one will notice you if you are practically hiding under the table!

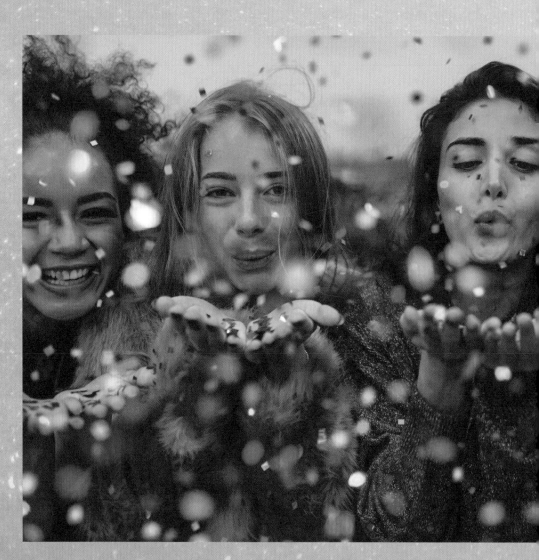

THE CHEERLEADER EFFECT

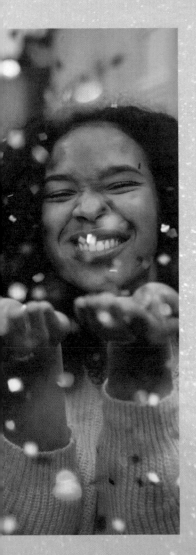

Just as being in a beautiful place or surrounding yourself with pretty objects can help to make you appear more attractive, so too can the people you associate with. A whole group of attractive people will understandably command more attention, and each individual will seem more attractive, because they have been accepted by their beautiful peers, so they too must be beautiful, right? This is known as the cheerleader effect, where the sum of the whole magnifies the perceived value of the individual, but it isn't only applied to women. Think about the collective attractiveness of a high-profile football team, where even an average-looking man suddenly becomes more of a catch due to the glamour attached to the team as a whole. The cheerleader effect can be very useful if you have a group of attractive friends to go out with. As a group, you will automatically attract significant amounts of attention, but if there is someone who catches your eye, be sure to step away from the group from time to time, so as not to be too intimidating to a potential new beau! Give them the space to approach you.

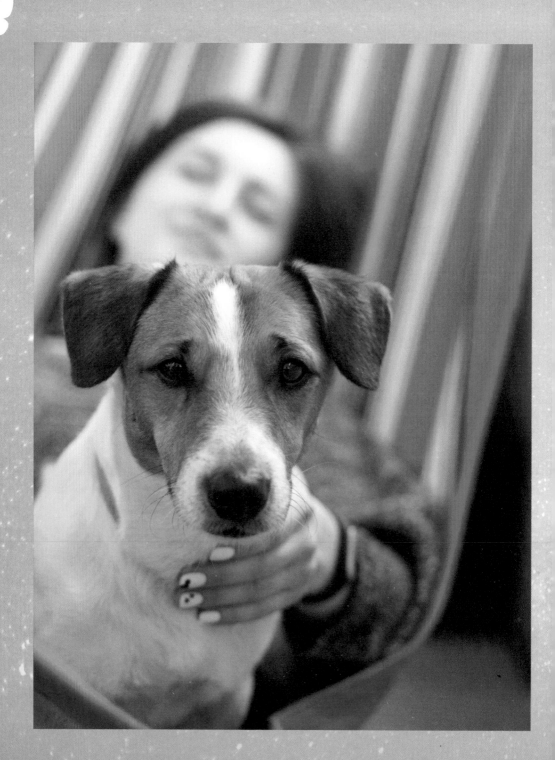

THE REPOUSSOIR

What if you don't have a large group of beautiful pals to hang out with? What else can you do to enhance your perceived attractiveness? Well, you could use the old French trick of finding a *repoussoir* – a word that comes from the world of fine art, meaning an object or person at the forefront of a painting. Such an object was designed to lead the viewer's eye towards the main subject and lend depth to the image.

In France, the matchmaking mothers of the 18th and 19th centuries took this idea one step further, hiring a real-life *repoussoir* – that is, a rather plain-looking young woman – to accompany their daughters out in society. In this way the *repoussoir* was thought to make the daughter look more attractive and therefore more marriageable.

So, you might like to think about being more strategic about whom you sit next to when you are out and about. Seating yourself next to a less attractive stranger on the bus, or in a café, will help to make you look more beautiful.

Alternatively, you could always get a dog. People have been subconsciously using dogs as *repoussoirs* for decades, as they know that pets can be a great way to meet prospective partners. The cute dog will draw the observer's eye straight to its owner – the perfect *repoussoir*!

ACCEPTING GIFTS

Glamorous people attract attention. They also attract small favours, compliments and little gifts. This is all part of living a glamorous life. There is no need to feel embarrassed. If someone gives you flowers or a small token of their appreciation, just smile and say thank you. You can always repay the favour when your admirer least expects it, perhaps when they are having a bad day. Accepting small favours isn't about taking advantage of anyone. It is simply a polite exchange of appreciation.

Small favours come in many guises: for example, the florist giving you the last bunch of roses before they wilt. The pâtissier adds an extra macaron because they know you have a particular favourite. A friend has a spare ticket to a concert and asks you to accompany them. All such favours might come your way when you start to work glamour magic.

Show gratitude and pass on the good vibes by offering to help someone else. The circulation of small favours and genuine compliments make the world a much more pleasant place to be. Knowing how to graciously give and receive is a very glamorous trait to have.

Glamourie: Attracting Gifts and Compliments

The best way to understand the power of glamour is to feel it for yourself. An unexpected gift or compliment is a sign that your glamour is on full display and the world is responding to that. To draw such favours into your life, light a tealight and hold your hands on either side, palms upwards to receive. Now say:

'Little gifts and pretty trinkets all come to me today
Compliments and shiny things are quick to come my way
As I go about my day, I enjoy a favoured life
As small favours find me, I pass them on to ease another's strife.'

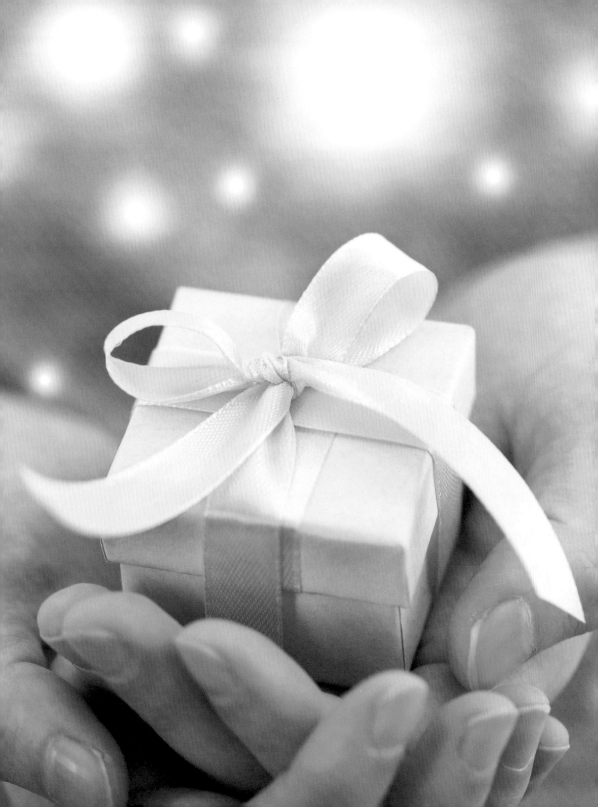

Chapter Three

Timeless Beauty

'*Beauty and femininity are ageless and can't be contrived...*'

MARILYN MONROE

Glamour is timeless, ageless and always in style. It has been ever-present throughout history and all eras have had their glamorous icons, from Cleopatra to Marie Antoinette, Grace Kelly to the Princess of Wales. Glamour is the stardust that gives certain people an ethereal glow that draws us in. We want a piece of their magic, which is why people flock to the cinema or to concerts to bask in the reflected light of their own personal idols.

There is no set age, weight or body type that makes someone glamorous: if you look back through history, we have glamorized all shapes and sizes at one time or another. Glamour isn't age-dependent, either. It isn't driven by trends and fashion – rather it is indefinable, that *je ne sais quoi* that the French talk about so much. But if you cannot clearly define it, how do you achieve it?

Glamour means different things to different people, but there are certain benchmarks that can help you to accomplish it. Avoiding trends is one. Think classic style over the latest fashions. Brand-chasing is another one to avoid. Designer labels should be subtle not showy. If you are not being sponsored to advertise a particular brand, why do it for free? Labels are much better on the inside of clothing, rather than emblazoned for all to see, which can come across as vulgar or crass.

Glamour is quiet, understated and elegant. It is almost a secret, a private little chat you have with yourself, but one with which society can also engage. Glamour is something you radiate. You never have to *tell* anyone that you are a high-value individual, that you deserve to be treated with respect or that you are worthy of the finer things in life. Your confidence, bearing and overall presentation will say all of this on your behalf. Just as you expect to pay a bit more in a fancy restaurant before you even look at the bill, so too will society pay you more regard and respect when you allow your glamour to shine through. When you value yourself, the rest will follow.

CREATE A GLAMOROUS BACKDROP

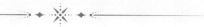

Beautiful people are drawn to beautiful things. They like to be surrounded with elegance and style, which is why glamorous people are drawn to glamorous places, such as Paris, New York, London and Rome. Glamorous people dine in fine restaurants, go shopping in the world's best department stores such as Harrods, Selfridges or Galeries Lafayette. They play glamorous sports, such as polo or dressage.

Of course, not everyone has the budget for such high levels of finery. In fact, most of us don't, but there are ways to bring the essence of these glamorous places into your life without robbing a bank to do so. If there is a particular place that immediately says 'glamour' to you, then begin to emulate it in your own home.

It might be that you can create a Parisian-themed apartment. Or perhaps you could try to recreate the dishes and cocktails from your favourite elite restaurants, which often publish their menus online. Maybe designing a Pegasus-themed dining room, with mirrored furniture and winged-horse ornaments, could recreate a taste of the Brasserie of Light, the chic Art Deco-themed restaurant in Selfridges, for instance. Whatever and wherever your ideal place of glamour is, use it as inspiration and bring the essence of it into your own home.

You don't have to spend a lot of money to do this. Just keep your eyes peeled for things that remind you of your favourite glamorous place and start to collect them for your home. You could go to thrift stores or antiques fairs to pick up bargains, or add a special little something to your Christmas wish list.

With a glamorous backdrop behind you, your personal glamour will automatically be elevated. Your home is your backdrop, your personal film set. It should reflect your dreams on a daily basis. It is the place to which you return after a busy day at work and it should feel like a place of escape – somewhere you can build the life you aspire to. It is the baseline for your glamorous journey, where you prepare yourself to go out into the world each day and where you cast your glamour spells to help you achieve your goals. Make sure it reflects the right energies so that you begin and end each day in a glamorous space.

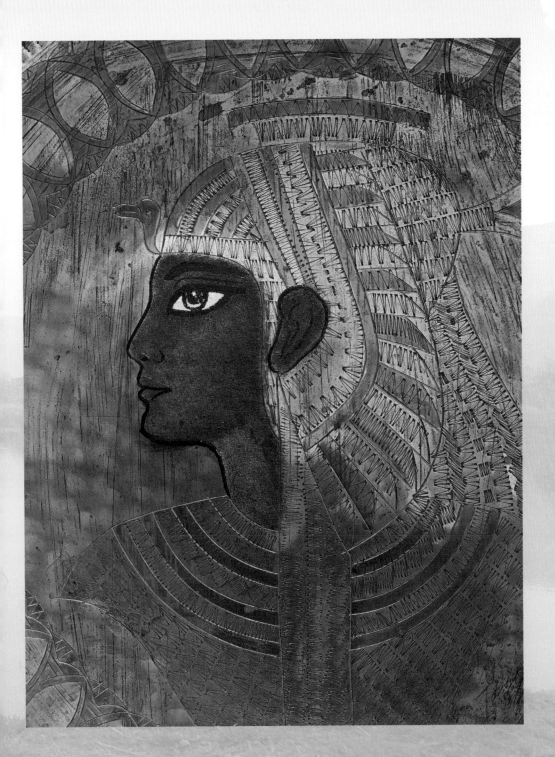

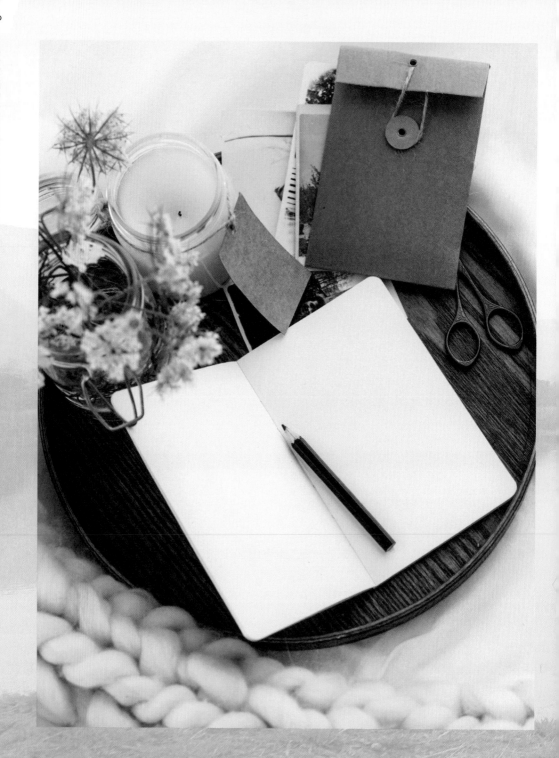

Glamourie: Design Your Personal Film Set

ITEMS REQUIRED: A notebook and pen, candles or incense.

Light the candles or incense and, to begin, sit quietly with your eyes closed and try to block out any distractions. Bring to mind an image of the most glamorous place you know. This could be somewhere you have visited in person, or a place you have read about or seen online. The important thing is that you feel a positive emotional connection to it.

Try to visualize the place in as much detail as possible, making the visualization as fully formed as it can be, engaging all of your senses. What does the place look like, what are the colours you see, how does the light fall? What are the scents, sounds and tastes? How tactile is it, what are the textures? What can you see? What ornamentation is around you? How does it make you feel emotionally and why are you drawn to it?

Now open your eyes and write down in your notebook everything that your visualization has just brought up, answering the questions posed above. When you are finished, you should have a detailed description of your perfect place of glamour. Read through what you have written. How do you feel as you do? Excited because you love to dream of it, or disheartened because you might never get there? Don't worry.

You are now going to begin the process of bringing the essence of that place into your daily life! Turn to a new page in the notebook and make a list of all the things your vision brought up – the colour, sound, smell, texture, taste and feelings. This list captures the essence of your most glamorous place and it can easily be recreated over time, by adding items from your list until eventually your home begins to resemble that glamorous location you dreamed about.

With the help of this list, you can carefully curate your belongings and your home so that they become the ideal backdrop to your glamorous life, just like a film set creates the right atmosphere for the actors to get into character and play out the scene. Your home is your own personal film set and it should set you up for the glamorous life you want to lead.

TIMELESS DÉCOR

Some aspects of home décor will always be considered glamorous, which is why elegant people are drawn to them, and why TV and magazine stylists always have them to hand. As I said earlier, being surrounded by beautiful things can make you appear more attractive. Here are some items that will help to create instant glamour in your home, whatever your budget.

- **Mirrors, mirrors, mirrors!** – There is a good reason why there's a saying about 'smoke and mirrors' – reflective surfaces can help to shine a light on the right spot, regardless of the season or time of day. Mirrors ensure that you are always bathed in natural light as much as possible. Use wall mirrors, reflective or mirrored furniture and full-length looking glasses to glam up your space. Art Deco, Art Nouveau, Venetian and classic arched mirrors are the most glamorous in design. It goes without saying that mirrors should always be spotless and gleaming for the best effects.

- **Candles** – The other half of the 'smoke and mirrors' adage, candles offer a flattering light. The flickering glow casts shadows around the room and over your features, softening sharp angles and lending an air of mystery. Scented candles add fragrance too, but ensure the room is well ventilated. Collect an assortment of candle holders to burn them safely and elegantly.

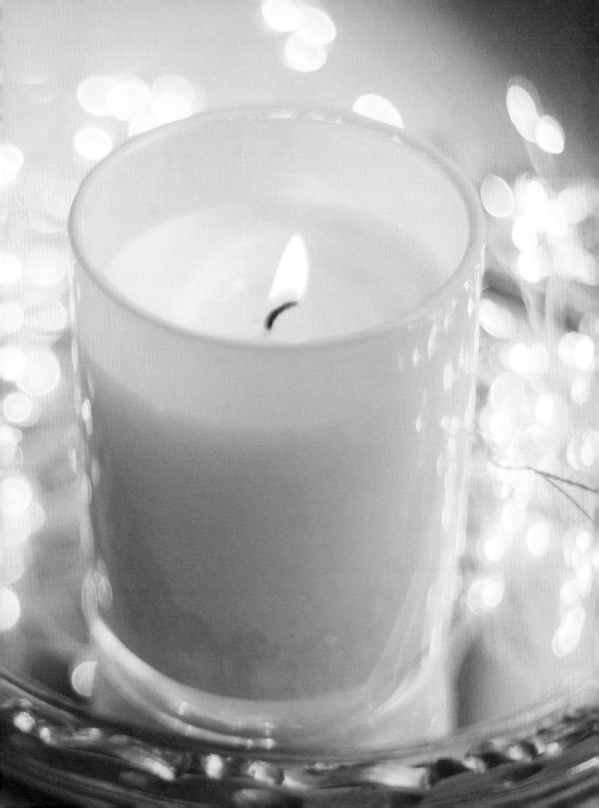

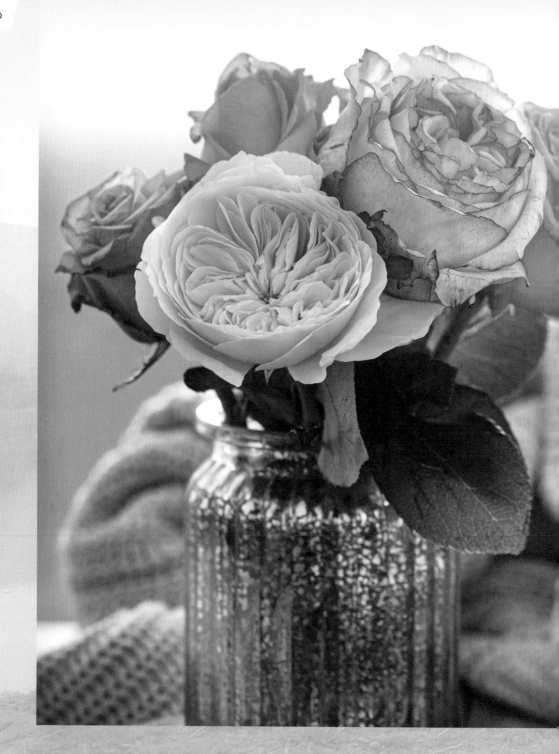

- **Flowers** – There is nothing like fresh flowers to brighten up any room – they add colour and a natural perfume to the space. They also make a statement, letting guests know that you care about your home and want to make it welcoming with fresh blooms. Having flowers around you will also make you seem more attractive (remember Anne Boleyn!) – especially when displayed in a mirrored or crystal vase.

- **Crystal** – There are two types of crystal that you can bring into your home to elevate the level of glamour. Natural crystals, such as pink quartz and amethyst, will imbue your home with earthly energies, helping to neutralize negative vibrations, while crystal tableware elevates the dining space. Cut or pressed glassware is a more affordable alternative to real crystal and it can be picked up piece by piece from antiques fairs and thrift shops. Like mirrors, crystal helps to bounce the light around and adds a touch of magic.

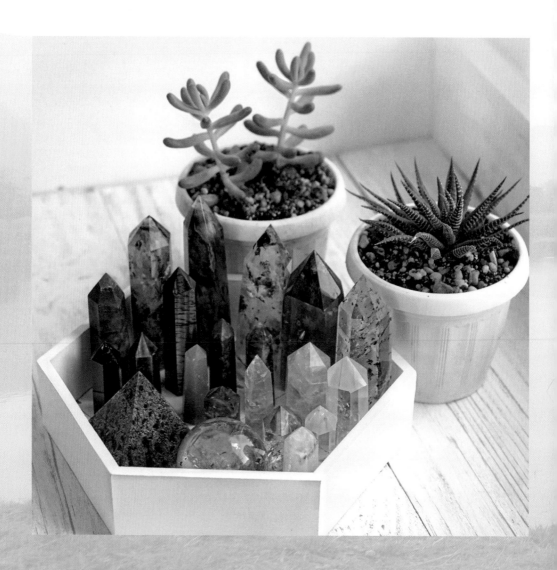

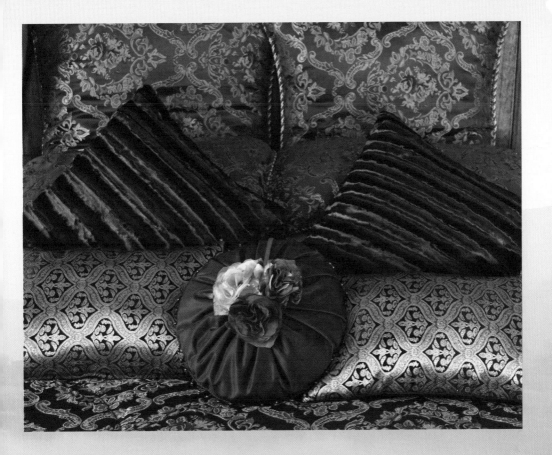

- **Plush fabrics** – Nothing says glamour like a bed or couch swathed in velvet, satin and brocade. Think velvet scatter cushions in jewel tones and thick tassels holding back floor-length curtains. Bed canopies, throws, cushions and faux furs can all add more glamour to a room.

Now that you have created a timeless and beautiful backdrop for the glamorous life you plan to lead, let's move on to developing your own personal idea of glamour and self-presentation.

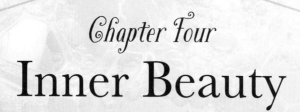

Chapter Four

Inner Beauty

'I don't try to be a sex-bomb. I am one!'

KYLIE MINOGUE

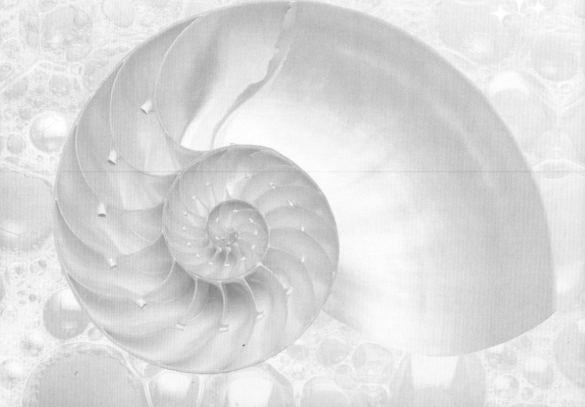

They say that beauty is in the eye of the beholder and, while there is some truth in this, it is also true that in order to be seen as beautiful, you must first of all begin to think of yourself that way. If you cannot see your own attractiveness, why expect anyone else to? Too often, people wait for permission from others to feel beautiful, but what if that permission never comes?

How you perceive yourself is half the battle. It is your own mind which sets the bar on how attractive you are. No one else can give you permission to feel pretty and, even if they did, how long would it be before you needed that validation again? This way of thinking creates a needy, clingy personality – someone who is always needing reassurance, which is exhausting for others to be around.

It is far better to take charge of your own attractiveness and to give yourself permission to feel beautiful. After all, no one else can give you a silent pep talk in the mirror when you need it, so why rely on anyone else? Besides, different people have different beauty standards and find different things attractive, so their opinions on your beauty will be just as varied. It is much better to set your own standard of beauty for yourself.

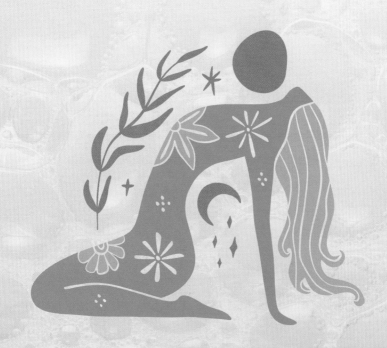

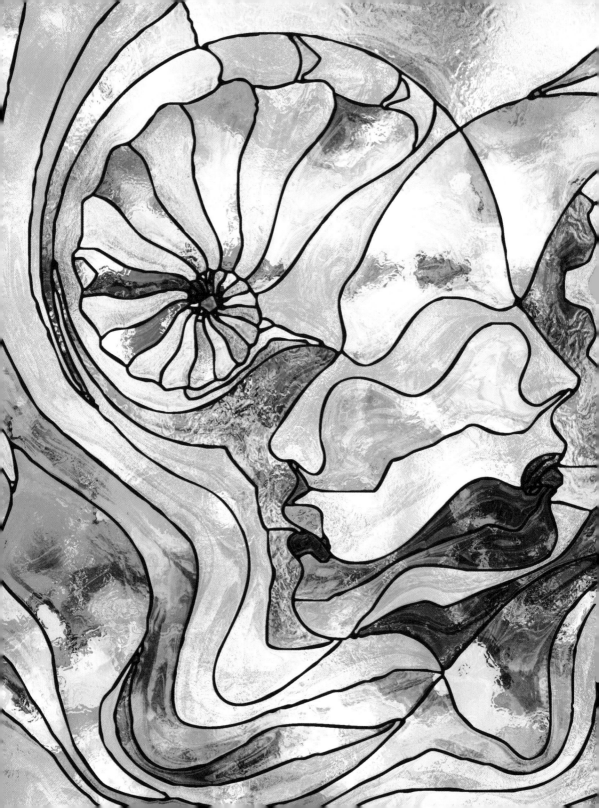

SET YOUR OWN BEAUTY STANDARD

Everyone has good points and bad points and none of us is perfect – not even supermodels. We all have insecurities. Glamour is about making the most of your best features, while playing down aspects of yourself that you think are less attractive. It's a personal decision.

Something else to consider is how natural you want your beauty to be, or not. You might draw the line at wearing false eyelashes, or having cosmetic procedures, or using fake tan. Then again you might prefer to use all the enhancements and tricks at your disposal! Again, this is your own personal beauty standard.

Bear in mind that just as fashions change, so, too, do the makeup trends and popular cosmetic procedures. We will be looking at makeup in more depth in Chapter Eight, but for now, suffice to say, that it is possible you might come to regret getting your eyebrows tattooed in blue ink, or your lips filled to the max, so always consider whether you are doing something for your own sake, or if it is because you have been influenced by trends.

In general, the more classic your look, the more timeless it's likely to be. Glamour isn't always bold and over the top – often it can be found in the little things; those small daily habits can make all the difference.

Glamourie: Your Makeup Manifesto

A manifesto is a declaration of your intentions – in this case, a declaration of what your minimum effort is going to be with regards to your beauty routine. This will be different for everyone. There is no one-size-fits-all approach. It will depend on your lifestyle and how much time you have available to prepare for the day. Your 'Makeup Manifesto' is your promise to yourself that this is the bare minimum you will do each and every day to help maximize your personal glamour. Your manifesto will be unique to you, but here are a few examples to get you started:

- I will never leave the house without at least applying lip gloss.
- I will cleanse, tone and moisturize every morning and evening.
- I will *always* remove my makeup at the end of each day, no excuses!
- I will use lovely products in the shower or bath each day – I will *not* stuff them in a drawer and save them for best!
- I will use a facemask once or twice a week.
- I will never leave the house without checking the mirror first.
- I will treat myself to a good makeup mirror.
- I will wear perfume every day, even if I'm not going anywhere.
  I will wear it for *me*.
- I will indulge in something glamorous every week – a candlelit bubble bath, a manicure, a facial – even if I do it myself at home.

You get the idea. Once you have decided on your personal manifesto, write it down and stick it in the bathroom or on your dressing-table mirror, where you can see it and be reminded each day of your commitment to yourself and your personal glamour.

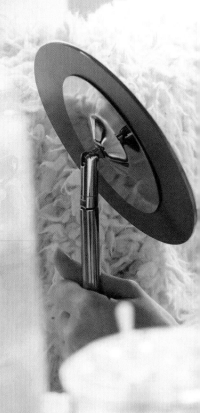

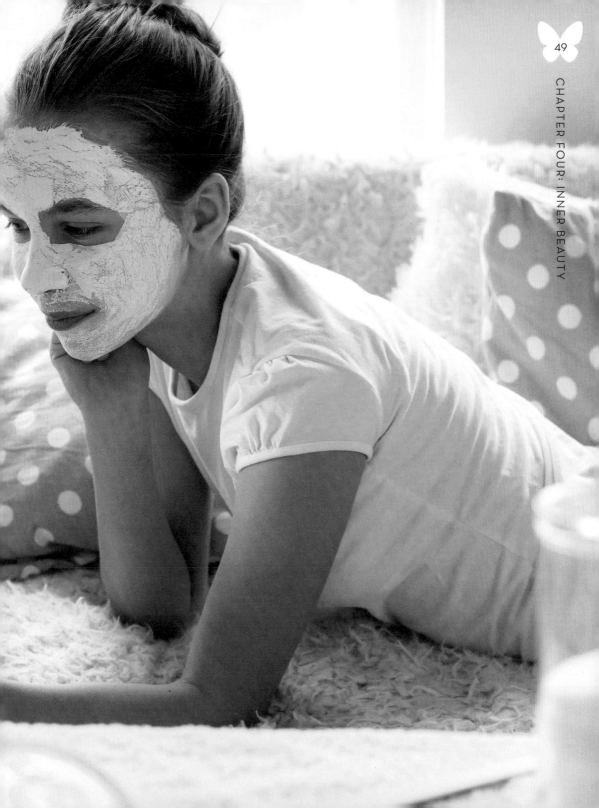

IT'S A QUEEN BEE STATE OF MIND

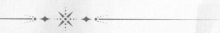

Becoming glamorous is about developing your queen bee mentality. Now this is not to say that you should begin to order people around and treat them like drones. No. It simply refers to the fact that you are playing the leading role in the story of your life, so you are, in effect, the queen bee – the one who is at the centre of it all. What you say goes. How you think, speak, act and present yourself will have an impact on how other people treat you. Treat yourself like a film star and those around you will follow suit.

If you permit someone to treat you badly, then you are unconsciously promoting that kind of behaviour towards yourself and they are likely to treat you badly again. What you permit, you promote. So, make sure that you stand strong in the face of rudeness and stare it down like a true queen bee.

Queen bee energy is great for increasing your confidence and resilience. You become bolder and ready to be seen. You get used to the buzz of people around you, trying to catch your eye or get your attention. It becomes natural for you to be the centre of attention, in a good way.

The opposite of queen bee energy is living apologetically, where you find yourself apologizing for everything, even your very existence! Someone bumps into you, for instance, and you say sorry to them. Or someone jumps the queue, stepping on your foot, and you apologize for not making room for them.

If you can relate to this, it is a habit you need to break by developing your queen bee mind-set instead. Own your space, don't apologize for it! You are the star of your own life, so take centre stage with confidence and pride. This is your curtain call to glamorous greatness!

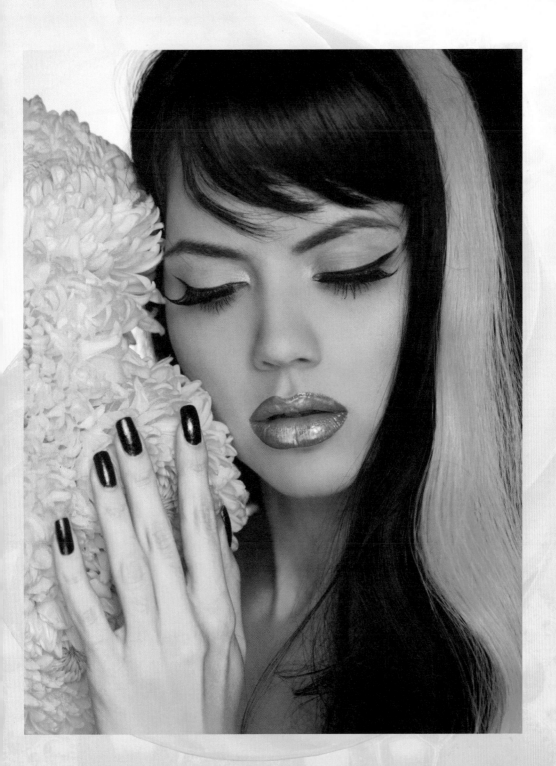

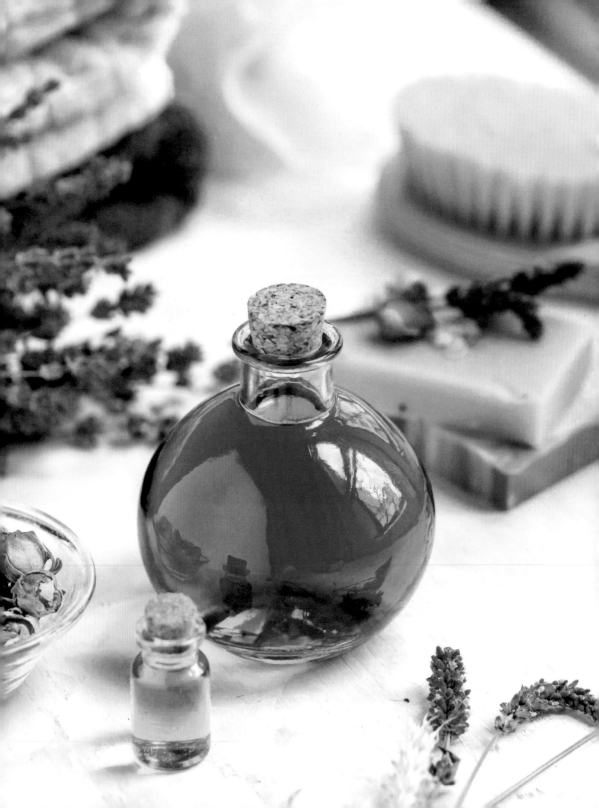

✦ Glamourie: Queen Bee Bathing Potion

ITEMS REQUIRED: You will need a jar of runny honey, rose or lavender essential oil, dried milk powder, candles for your bathroom.

Never underestimate the power of honey in your beauty routine. As a natural antioxidant it works wonders for your skin, drawing out impurities and leaving it feeling soft and silky. Honey also has antibacterial properties, so it is good for soothing minor skin irritations too. Cleopatra knew the beauty benefits of honey, so take a tip from her and bathe in milk and honey, using the following bath potion.

- Take a large jug and pour in one pint of hot water.
- Add three tablespoons of runny honey and stir until it has dissolved into the water.
- Add six drops of rose or lavender essential oil.
- Run a bath and add three tablespoons of dried milk powder to it. Stir with your hands until it dissolves.
- Finally pour in the contents of the jug and stir the water until it is evenly mixed.
- Light some candles and bathe like an ancient queen bee!

GLAM-O-METER

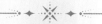

Different situations call for different degrees of glamour. Think of glamour as being on a dial, like a thermostat. Sometimes you will need to turn it up high, while, on other occasions, it will serve you better to turn it down a notch. Just as you wouldn't wear a ballgown to a funeral, so you shouldn't head into a job interview exuding the same degree of glamour as you would on a date. So how do you decide how glamorous you need to be? It depends on the situation.

Imagine your glam-o-meter as a dial, which is divided into sections: low, medium and high. Low means that you are polished and well turned out, but not in any way seductive. Medium means that you can dress less conservatively, but your interactions are no more than friendly conversations and a building of rapport.

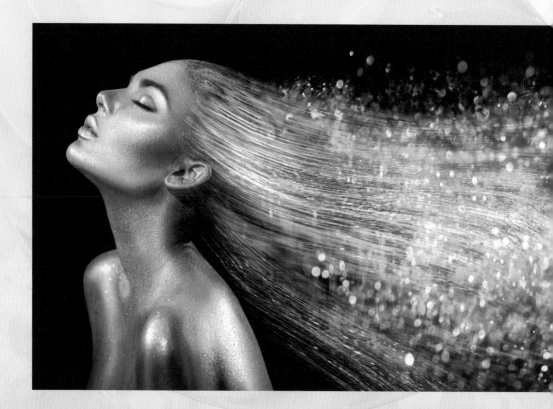

High means that you are in full seduction or performance mode and you can be as glamorous and flamboyant as you choose. You can attribute any occasion to one of these sections so that you know how much glamour to deploy, for example:

- **Low glam** – A funeral, religious ceremony, medical appointment, legal meeting, court appearance or jury duty.
- **Medium glam** – A job interview, promotion or performance review, hen party, baby shower, garden party, barbecue, graduation, business lunch, networking event or seminar, relaxed holiday, shopping trip, pop concert, book signing or audition.
- **High glam** – A day at the races, wedding, engagement party, birthday or festive occasion, ballet, opera, classical concert, country house party or date night.

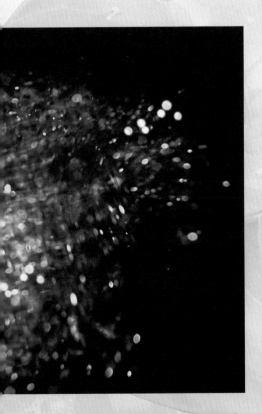

As soon as you receive an invitation to an event, begin to ask yourself where that event might fall on the glam-o-meter. Then you can begin to prepare accordingly, choosing the most appropriate outfit and makeup look for that occasion. Don't be afraid to dial your personal glamour up and down, as the need dictates. It isn't meant to be static – it should fluctuate and flow in accordance with the situations you find yourself in. Not only does this kind of mental preparation instil you with greater social confidence, it can also save you from an unfortunate *faux pas*. No one wants to see your gold Madonna-style corset at a baby's christening!

Chapter Five
It's a Mystery

'Very few of us are
what we seem.'

AGATHA CHRISTIE

An air of mystery is one of the key components of glamour, but in an age in which people document their lives on the internet, it can be very difficult to cultivate it. Mystery is enticing. It attracts interest in the same way a flame attracts moths, and mystery and glamour go hand in black-velvet-glove.

Just like at a masquerade ball, where everyone wears a mask to hide part of their face and no one can ever be quite sure with whom they are dancing, a little mystique can make you far more alluring. Think of the romantic appeal, on the silver screen, of highwaymen, or characters such as Zorro, the Lone Ranger and the Phantom of the Opera, to name but a few – all of whom use the mystery of hidden identity to draw people into their sphere, for good or ill.

In the modern world, it could be said that the internet provides a digital mask for people to wear. After all, you can never be entirely sure whom you are interacting with online, or if they are all that they claim to be. It is easy to hide on the internet; it is easy to pretend to be someone else. The mask of a social media platform is frequently used to create the illusion of a more glamorous life, with people offering a highlight reel of their week, skipping out all the boring parts, the inconveniences and setbacks, to give the impression that they live more glamorously than they actually do. No one ever posts pictures of themselves putting the bins out in their dressing gown and slippers, do they? Remember that if scrolling through social media leaves you feeling a little deflated, because much of what you are consuming online is no more than other people's carefully crafted highlights.

LIFE IS A MASQUERADE BALL

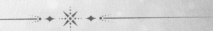

Figuratively speaking, we all wear masks from time to time. It is one of our survival skills. You might smile when you are down in the dumps, or laugh and make jokes from a hospital bed to disguise the fact that you are in pain. You might talk about putting on a brave face when feeling scared, or putting your face on when applying makeup. Masks are just a part of life, but whether it's one of comedy or tragedy is largely your own choice.

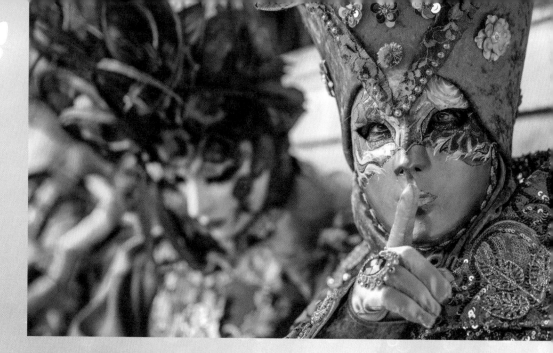

The truth is that day-to-day life is something of a masquerade ball. You never truly know what someone is going through or what mask they wear to hide it. The life and soul of the office party might be suffering from depression, for instance. The woman who, on the surface, seems to have her life in total control might be struggling behind closed doors. You just never know, so it is always wisest to assume that everyone has their own issues and to be kind to other people and give them the benefit of the doubt.

Masks are a great defence mechanism. They are one of the ways people keep going through difficult times. Usually, the masks people wear tend to be subconscious – they don't know they are covering up; they only know that they feel safer when they present themselves a certain way. Ripping away someone's mask means robbing them of their security and they might never forgive you for it. Generally speaking, the metaphorical mask will only come off when the individual is ready to set it aside and show their true face, not before.

How does all this connect with glamour and mystery? Well, if people wear masks all the time anyway, you might as well take the time to cultivate your own mask on a more conscious level, creating one that exudes confidence, allure and magnetism. And yes, a little bit of mystery too.

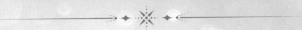

VENETIAN MASQUERADE MAGIC

The mask is a great metaphor for self-styling. It is the embodiment of 'fake it till you make it.' Comedy or tragedy, hero or villain, wealthy or poor, transparent or mysterious – the choice is always yours, so choose the mask you wear each day very carefully.

When people think of masks, the city of Venice often springs to mind. The Venice Carnival dates back to the 13th century and it still takes place each year in February. It is a ten-day event of masked pageants, processions and balls. The colours of the masks are symbolic, conveying a message to fellow guests without having to reveal oneself or say a word.

- **White** signifies virtue, purity, virginity and youth.
- **Gold** signifies royalty, acquired wealth, status, illumination, enlightenment, divine masculine energies, wisdom and prestige.
- **Silver** signifies nobility, ambition, intelligence, wealth-building, elevation and divine feminine energies.
- **Red** signifies sexuality, power, control, dominance, risk-taking and high energy.
- **Pink** signifies sensuality, femininity, gentleness, softness, kindness and good health.
- **Purple** signifies magic, enchantment, creativity, science, alchemy and psychic energy.
- **Blue** signifies constancy, truth, loyalty, tranquillity, even temper, trust and faithfulness.
- **Green** signifies fertility, growth, confidence, grounded energy, strength, stamina and longevity.
- **Orange** signifies action, proactive energy, communication, courage, flamboyance, sociability, enthusiasm, happiness, success, achievement and good humour.
- **Black** signifies sophistication, elegance, authority, status, dignity, mystery, seduction, sadness, tragedy, sexual power play, control and contrivance.

✦ Glamourie: Create Your Mask of Mystery

Having a visual representation of what you want to convey can be very helpful, so in this exercise you are going to create your own Venetian-style mask. You can buy blank masks from crafts stores or online. Use whatever you like to decorate yours – paints, felt-tip pens, glitter, fabrics, feathers and so on.

Using the colour magic list above, decide what kind of mask you are going to create. This mask will represent your own personal glamour and mystery. If you are naturally flamboyant, you might want to lean towards the darker colours to bring out your more mysterious side, for example. On the other hand, if you are very shy and struggle to be seen, then use the metallic shades, with a dash of red or purple. Whatever way you choose to design and decorate your mask is fine – there is no right or wrong way to do this, so have fun with it. Once you have finished decorating your mask and all the paint, glue and decorations are completely dry, hold it in your hands to empower it and say:

This mask shows who I wish to be
A person of glamour and mystery
A creature of unfettered grace
Now comes across in my true face
As this magic mask stares down at me
It reminds me of who I'm meant to be!'

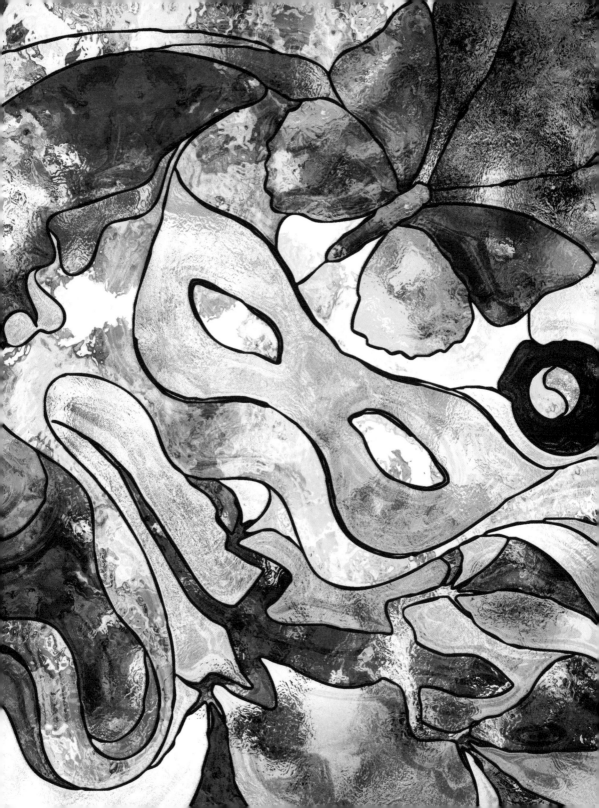

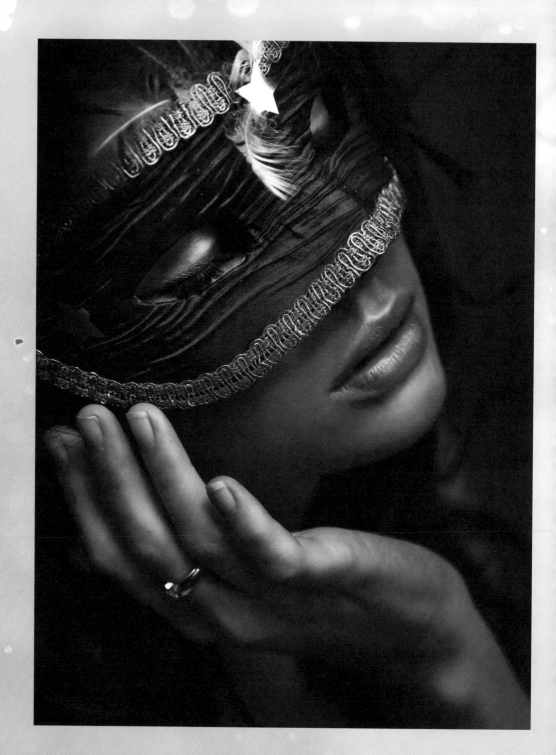

Put on the mask and wear it for a few minutes. Look at yourself in the mirror. Imagine that you are seeing yourself for the first time, a stranger in the mask. What is your first thought? Do you find the person in the mirror mysterious, glamorous, contrived, fun? How do you feel with this mask covering your face? Are you happy to hide away or do you like the mask you have created so much that you wish you could wear it all the time? This mask represents the hidden side of yourself – the one you don't show very often. When you feel ready, take off the mask, but place it somewhere you will see it often, so that it can remind you of who you aim to be.

DRAWING DOWN THE VEIL: BECOMING MORE MYSTERIOUS

Being mysterious is like drawing a veil over certain aspects of your life. They are not hidden, but nor are they on full display for all to see. Developing an air of mystery can be an ongoing process and some people find it more difficult than others. In general, if you are a naturally quiet person, then being mysterious should be easier because you are not in the habit of chatting away to everyone you meet. However, if you tend to overshare and tell everyone about your personal life, then cultivating an air of mystery will be somewhat harder.

Why do we need to be mysterious? Because we live in a world where there is too much information circulating and where we are conditioned into believing that we should always be transparent on everything, to everyone, at all times. Nothing could be further from the truth. No one is entitled to know everything there is to know about you – and there are some things that should be kept to yourself. Sensitive topics should not be discussed with people you have just met, so you might like to consider keeping your opinions on religion, politics and so forth to yourself when you first meet people. The same goes for any current, contentious topics too.

Being mysterious also gives people a chance to get to know you slowly, over a period of time. It means that they will learn to trust you more quickly too, because they will see that you are not in the habit of repeating everything you hear. Your conversation is cordial and discreet, not gossipy and sensationalist. Here are a few tips to help you bring more mystery to your personality and interactions:

- Speak less – listen more. Show greater interest in the person you are talking to, so that you give away less information about yourself.
- Be careful what you share on social media. Book recommendations or mentioning a great play you saw at the theatre is fine, but save the true confessions for the confessional!
- Take a break from social media, but don't give any warning of it. Just disappear from all your platforms for a time. No likes, no posts, no comments – nothing. This is very good for your mental health and it will keep everyone guessing!
- Let people wonder what you're doing. You don't have to tell them everything.
- Don't just *act* busy – *be* busy. Build a life you love and fill it with hobbies and adventures.
- Have a secret hobby or interest that no one else knows about and indulge in it frequently.

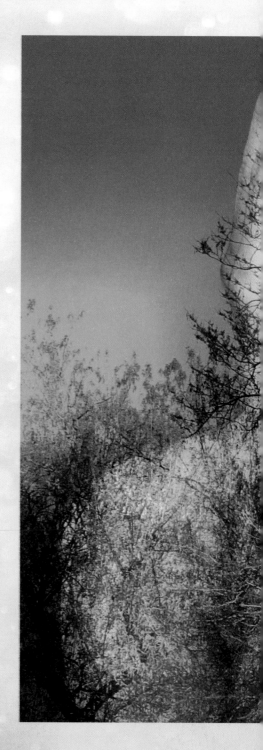

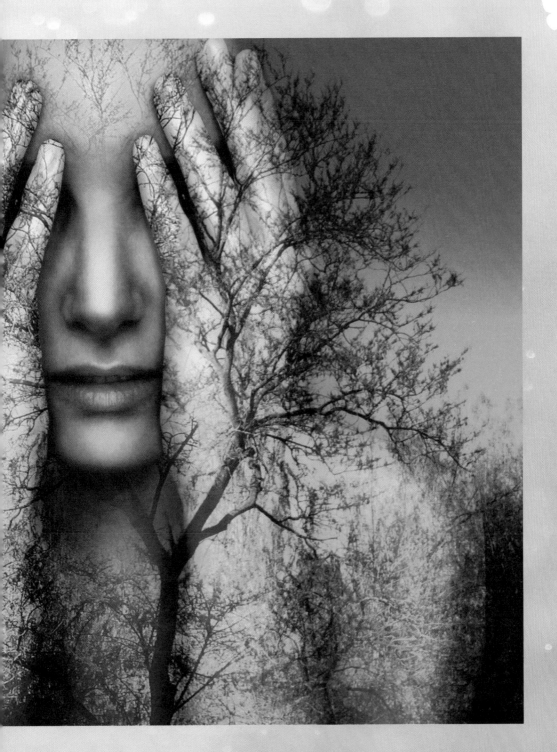

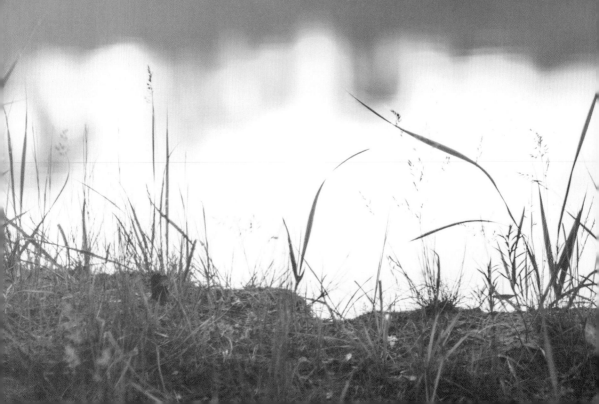

- Have a secret little place you go to. Just you. It could be a place in the countryside, a little pub or café, a bench in a beautiful park. But find a place of your own and keep it to yourself.
- Keep your shopping habits to yourself, unless you want the people you know to go and buy all the same things as you! Don't give away details

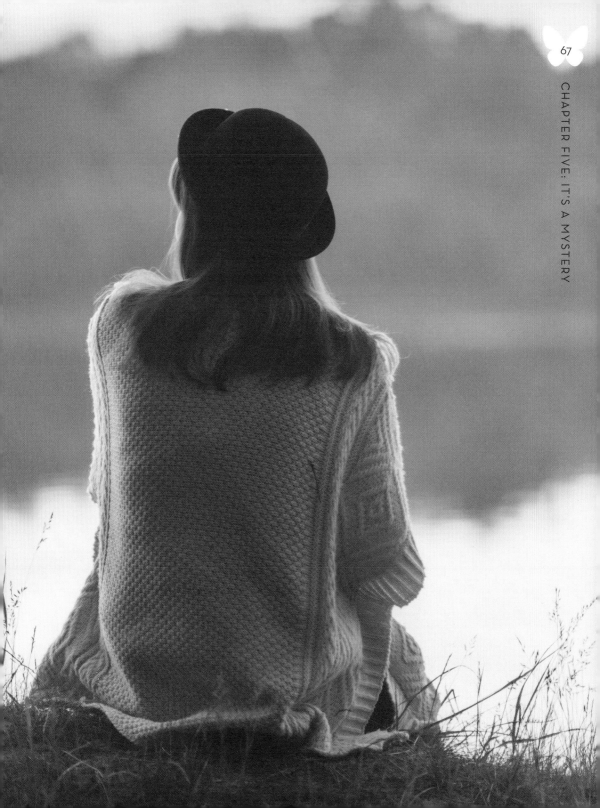

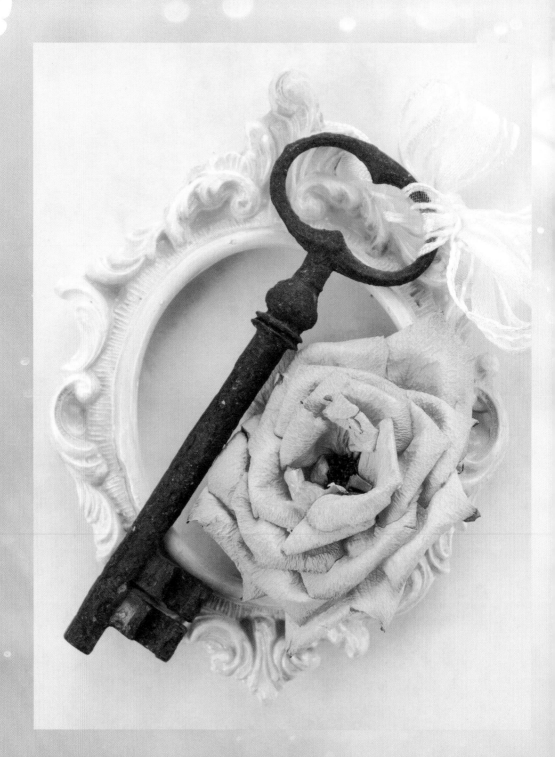

of your favourite boutique, or where you get your hair done. Protect your style with a little mystery about its origins.

- When questioned, respond vaguely then change the subject or create a pleasant distraction.
- Be independent. Do things alone and often.
- Smile to yourself in public, as if you have a delicious secret. People will wonder what you're smiling about.
- Keep your personal life private. No one needs to know how many partners you've had or where you buy your underwear.
- Wear sunglasses, especially mirrored ones – hiding the eyes is very mysterious.
- Attend a masquerade ball whenever you can!

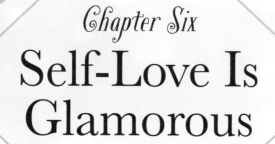

Chapter Six
Self-Love Is Glamorous

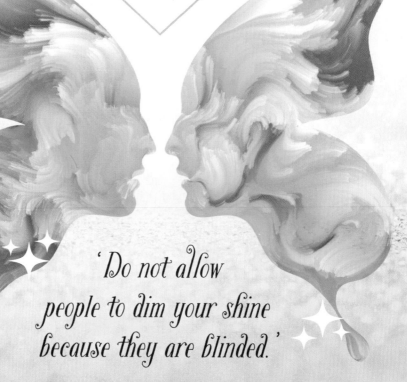

'Do not allow
people to dim your shine
because they are blinded.'

LADY GAGA

Nothing is more glamorous than a person who knows how to value and take care of themselves. This goes far beyond good grooming – it includes such skills as graciously making yourself less available and knowing your worth in relationships and the workplace, as well as keeping up standards of appearance. You don't only *look* glamorous, or live a glamorous lifestyle, you exude glamour in your interactions and intentions towards yourself too. If you accept shabby treatment, then people will treat you in a shabby way. You must first elevate how you treat yourself and other people, if you want the world to respond in kind.

Self-love is all about how you see yourself and how you view your place in the world. It is the opposite of having low self-esteem and not feeling good enough. When you have a high level of love for yourself, you will naturally feel that you deserve to be treated well. Practices such as having good manners, being kind to others and treating people in a gracious and kindly way will lead to the energies that you send out into the world being reflected back to you.

IMPOSTER SYNDROME

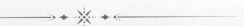

Have you ever felt like you don't belong or that you are not worthy of your current situation? Imposter syndrome happens to most of us from time to time. You might feel like you didn't really deserve to get that big promotion at work, or that you don't belong in a high-end restaurant or glamorous department store, or even that you are unworthy of your partner. Signs of imposter syndrome include:

- Telling yourself that you are not good enough for something.
- Thinking or muttering, 'I don't belong here!'
- Believing that you don't deserve the good things in life.
- Imagining that you might be escorted from the building because you're a fraud.
- Thinking that other people will see right through you.
- Feeling as if you are about to be 'found out' as an imposter or phony.
- Believing that your success is all down to luck.

- Fearing that you will be a disappointment or that you won't be able to live up to expectations.
- Having so much self-doubt that you cannot strategize or move your life forward.
- Refusing opportunities and invitations because you think they have been offered to you by mistake or out of politeness.
- Existing in a constant state of stage-fright.
- Consistently questioning your own abilities and intelligence.

Imposter syndrome is the opposite of glamour and it can derail all your plans to live a confident, glamorous life. Interestingly, people who have experienced poverty, or who come from a humble background, tend to suffer more from imposter syndrome than those with greater affluence, although it can affect anyone. This could be because less well-off people rarely get the opportunity to experience significant wealth and the glamour that naturally accompanies richer surroundings, leading them to believe that such things are not meant for them.

Overcoming imposter syndrome is largely a mental battle. You must tell yourself repeatedly that you *are* good enough and deserving of all the wonderful opportunities that life sends your way, then grab onto them with both hands and enjoy your good fortune. In the meantime, you can use the following ritual to help you deal with self-doubt. Remember that glamour spells are about shifting the perspective, not only of how others see you, but also how you see yourself too. Self-love means that your glam-o-meter should be set at a medium level.

✦ Glamourie: Lavender Scrub to Slough off Self-Doubt

ITEMS REQUIRED: You will need a mixing bowl, wooden spoon, half a cup of sea salt, almond oil, lavender essential oil, dried lavender, an empty jar and lid.

In a bowl, mix the sea salt with enough almond oil to make a thick paste. Add two or three teaspoons of dried lavender and mix it in thoroughly. Next, add between five and 10 drops of lavender oil, depending on how strong you want the fragrance to be, and stir it in. Once the paste is thoroughly mixed together, transfer it to the jar and put on the lid. Use as a body scrub next time you shower. As you do so, imagine that you are scrubbing away the imposter syndrome that holds you back. Shed the dead skin of self-doubt and step out of the shower with a glamorous glow that enables you to take on the world!

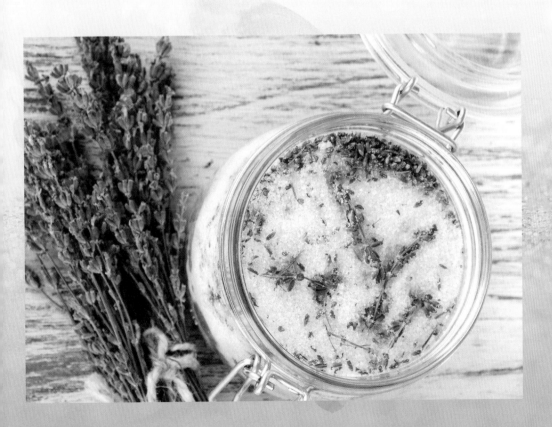

BEWARE OF SELF-SLIGHTING

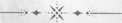

Self-slighting is when you treat yourself in an inferior way to how you treat other people. It is one of those things that is so subtle you don't always know you're doing it. It manifests in small, seemingly insignificant ways, but they all add up to a bad habit. Here are some of the ways you might slight yourself in day-to-day life:

- Saving the best tea and coffee for guests, while using an inferior brand yourself.
- Eating burnt toast and making fresh toast for your kids or partner.
- Saving things for best – you deserve to use them now!
- Answering the front door to guests, but using the back door yourself. The back door was once the tradesman's entrance, so using this entrance implies that you are not worthy of living in your own home!
- Not bothering to set a nice dinner table when you eat alone.
- Not bothering to cook for yourself because you believe it's not worth cooking for one.
- Having a quick shower when you really want a long, luxurious bath.
- Not taking care of yourself or 'letting yourself go'.

Self-slighting is very common and it is easily remedied. Simply begin to treat yourself as you would a guest. Make sure that you are using all your nice things: light those fancy candles, lay the table with the best china and glassware, open that bottle of wine, wear your pretty jewellery or best ties. Treat yourself like a film star and others will soon follow suit. This is the key to a glamorous lifestyle.

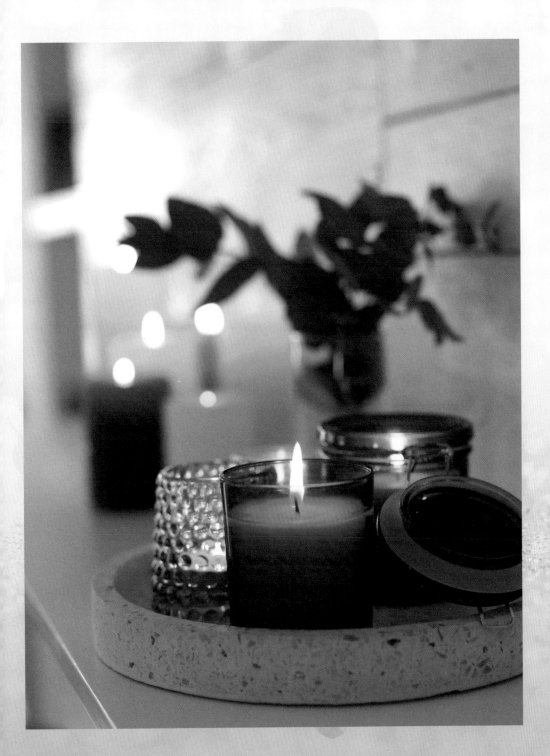

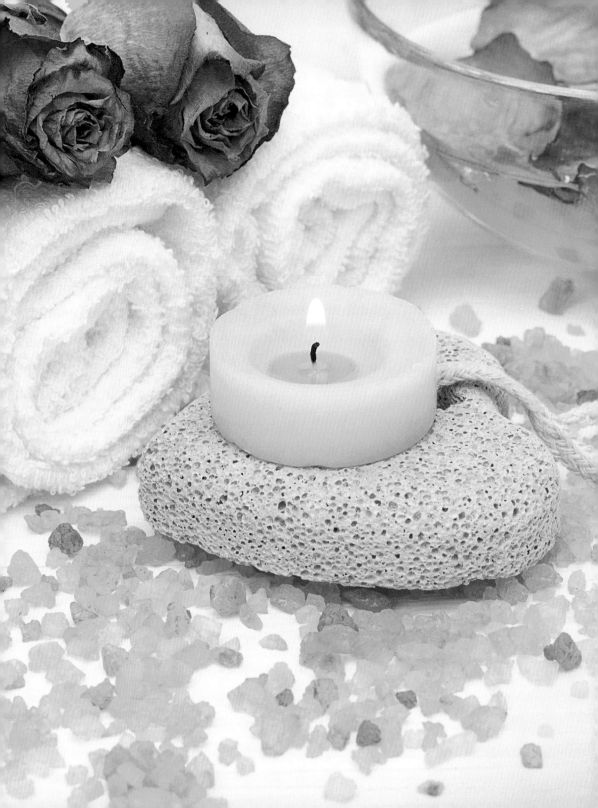

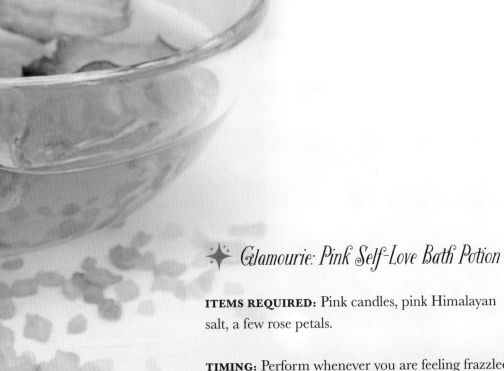

✦ *Glamourie: Pink Self-Love Bath Potion*

ITEMS REQUIRED: Pink candles, pink Himalayan salt, a few rose petals.

TIMING: Perform whenever you are feeling frazzled.

There will be days when you feel that you cannot do anything right, when you feel like you've been running late since the moment you woke up and one mishap leads straight into another, leaving you feeling stressed and decidedly frazzled. On those days, show yourself some love with this bath potion. Mix together equal parts pink Himalayan salt and rose petals, then stir this mixture into a hot bath. The salt is known to reduce fatigue and help with emotional balance, while the rose petals will soften the skin as the fragrance uplifts you. Wallow in the water for as long as you comfortably can, then dry off and allow your troubles to go down the drain, ensuring that you dispose of the rose petals on the compost heap. Enhance this ritual by using rose-scented toiletries.

BE GRACIOUSLY INACCESSIBLE

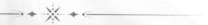

Glamorous people tend to be quite elusive. They do not overstay their welcome anywhere, nor do they accept every invitation. Part of their charm is that they make themselves so rare. Spending an hour or two in their company feels like a precious gift – and it is, because there is nothing more valuable than time, so be careful how much of *your* time you give away to others. Your career, family and close friends will naturally have the lion's share of your time, but the hours and days you have

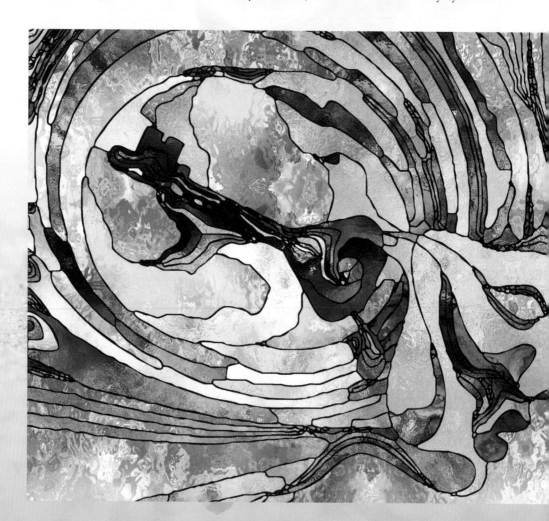

left to spare should be guarded carefully. This is because there are those people who will siphon off your time and energy if you allow them to, leaving you feeling drained and exhausted. No matter how many hours of the day you give to them, they will always want more. It will never be enough. Watch out for this, because as you become more glamorous and confident, you will also become more magnetic to others and you will inevitably attract those individuals who want to fill themselves up with your energy. Don't let them. Set your boundaries and use these tips to become as elusive as a butterfly. Catching you should feel like trying to hold onto Scotch mist!

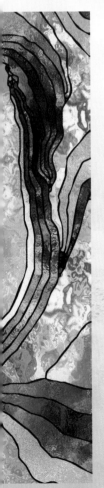

- Think of yourself as an elusive creature of mystery.
- Set time aside for solitude – rest, read, pamper and relax.
- Keep your activity schedule private to avoid being gate-crashed.
- Switch off your phone and enjoy silence for an hour or two.
- Screen your calls – this means that you can avoid time-wasting phone calls about nothing from long-winded acquaintances. Or from unsuitable suitors too, for that matter!
- Understand what your time is worth and how much an event will cost you in terms of time and energy spent, because you will never get it back.
- Graciously refuse any invitation that you really don't want to attend. No event should feel like an obligation, not even your niece's nativity play!
- Remember that an early night, in bed with a good book, is a social engagement with yourself and not one that should be cancelled.
- For the sake of sanity, make relaxing social engagements with yourself regularly and often!

BEWARE THE CINDERELLA COMPLEX

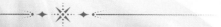

Do you have a Cinderella complex, where you are constantly running around doing things for others, with no time left to yourself? Do you feel undermined, undervalued and put upon? If so, this is an act of self-sabotage, *not* self-love! Helping out family members or doing the occasional favour for a friend is one thing, but if you find yourself constantly being asked for assistance from all and sundry, then this is a sign that you are a bit of a soft touch and you need to learn how to set stronger boundaries, even saying no occasionally.

Ask yourself if the person who is requesting the favour could easily do the task themselves. If they could, then it is likely that they are taking advantage of your good nature. What are their motivations for asking you to do the task for them? Are they trying to put you in your place, pull rank or subtly belittle you?

Are you genuinely being invited to a party, for instance, or are you simply being allowed to stay after you have prepared all the food? There is a significant difference here. The first respects you as an honoured guest, while the second condescends to you as an inferior servant who is offered the crumbs from the table. You must learn how to make this type of distinction and recognize when someone is behaving condescendingly towards you.

If you feel like a ragged, overworked Cinderella, then the chances are that you are in the company of an Ugly Stepsister or two. Don't put up with it. Stand up for yourself instead, by graciously refusing the invitation. Let the Ugly Stepsisters make their own buffet – you have a far more glamorous and successful life to lead!

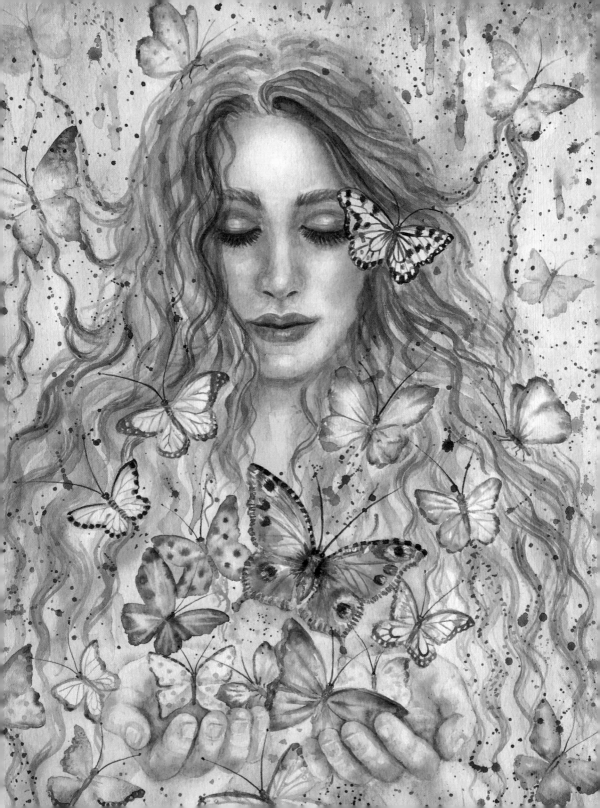

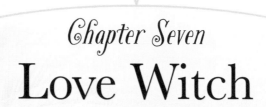

Chapter Seven
Love Witch

'*How do I love thee? Let me count the ways.*'

ELIZABETH BARRETT BROWNING

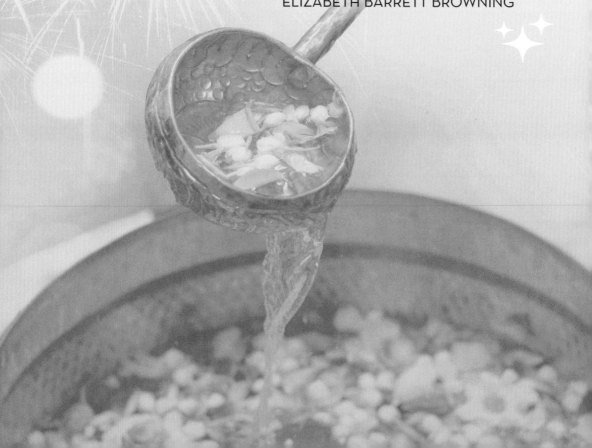

There is no doubt that being more glamorous can improve your love life. This is because the first seeds of attraction are sown at a physical level. You have to be able to catch someone's eye and hold their attention, just as they need to be able to hold your attention too. A physical attraction is the very first step on the path to love and romance, so without it you won't get very far. Fortunately, we are all attracted to different things, so you don't need film-star looks to attract a new love into your life. There is someone for everyone and glamour magic can draw them to you.

Love magic is a way to enhance your own sex appeal. It is not designed to force a specific person to fall in love with you. Instead, it is meant to create a magnetic field of allure around you, so that you naturally receive much more attention. You can then decide if you want to accept such attention and take the relationship further.

Glamour can also enhance an existing relationship. Making the most of your best features and wearing nicer outfits can help to rekindle the romance in a long-term partnership. A new haircut can make your spouse look at you quite differently. If you're not ready for a new hair-do, think about adding to your allure with accessories that have sex appeal – for instance, a pair of black leather gloves, or a new fragrance.

Love magic is especially dependent upon emotions, for there is no greater feeling than that of love. There is no drug or adrenaline-junkie experience that can compare with the feeling of falling in love with someone you think is wonderful – and they don't call it *falling* in love for no reason. Love frequently takes us completely by surprise, coming along when we least expect it and leading to a headlong stumble into a relationship. The fall can be amazing – providing that the object of your desires is there to catch you. Unrequited love is a painful experience, yet the love itself is real enough – it just isn't being reciprocated. And then, of course, there is heartbreak, brought about by betrayal, loss or by a lover who simply changed their mind, as people are wont to do.

Love is amazing, exhilarating, confusing, infuriating and frustrating. At times, it can be a lonely experience too. It is nevertheless a road that we must all navigate in our lives, often more than once, so having glamour magic on your side to help smooth out the bumps in the road to true romance can only be a good thing!

✦ Glamourie: Step into Your Magnetic Persona

Glamour is about perception. It is an illusion cast to help others see you in the most flattering way. All spells that cover beauty and confidence are effective glamour spells, but, for casting love spells specifically, we need to ramp up the glamour even more. Creating a persona is a good way to increase your magnetism, drawing people into your orbit by the power of a glamorous aura. To begin, you will need to come up with a persona that is everything you believe a glamorous person would be. You can use fictional characters, film stars or singers as your inspiration – whoever you admire and aspire to emulate.

Create this character in your mind's eye. What do they look like, what kind of clothes do they wear, what is their signature fragrance? Visualize this character as clearly as you can and imagine the kind of suitors and positive attention they attract wherever they go. If it helps to draw or write about this persona, then by all means do so. It needs to be as clear as possible to you. Visualize this character standing in front of you, then simply step into that persona and say:

'A glamorous new me is set free this day
This new persona now takes flight
As I become who I'm meant to be
I shimmer in glamorous light
All who see me are drawn my way
A true beauty they shall see
This glamour is cast with each new day
As I learn to live out the new me!'

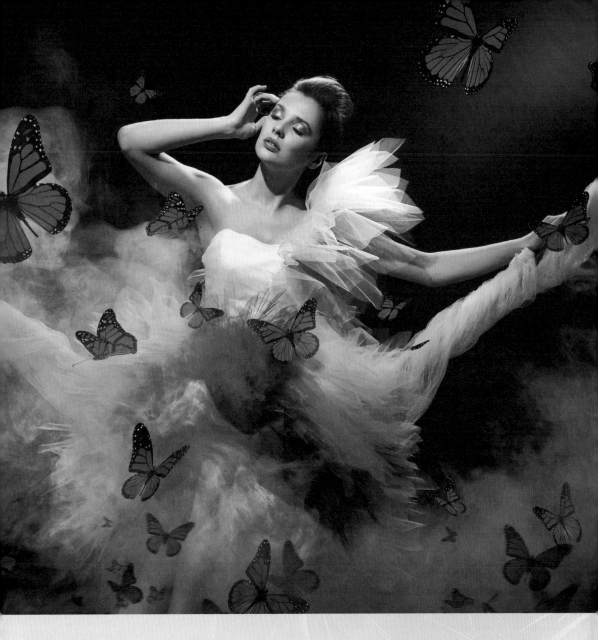

Activate this glamour spell each time you want to draw more positive attention your way. It is great for parties, dates and generally going about your day, exuding a glamorous magnetism wherever you go. It always a good glamourie to cast before the following love spells, to give yourself the best chances of success.

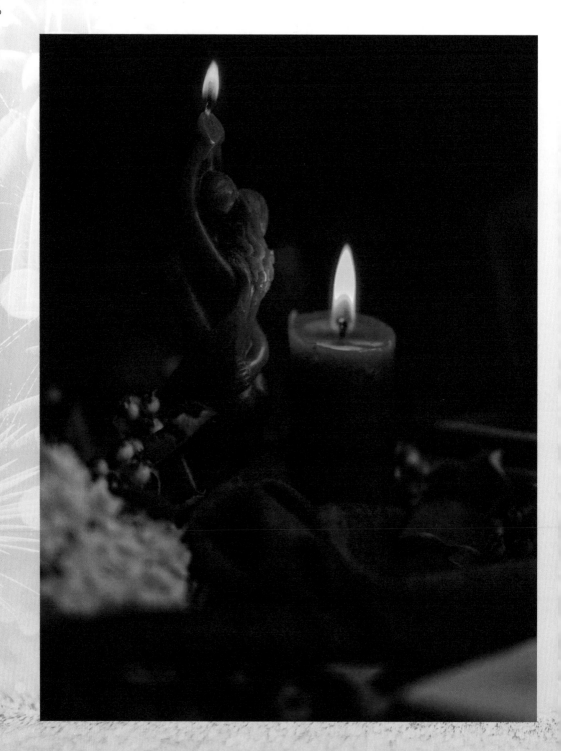

✦ Glamourie: Three Moons Spell to Attract Love

ITEMS REQUIRED: Three red candles, half a teaspoon of blessing seeds, mortar and pestle, kitchen roll, rose or lavender oil, athame or carving tool, cauldron or heatproof bowl, lighter.

TIMING: Perform on the full moon, three months in a row.

Take one of the candles and carve what you are hoping to attract into the length of the wax, so you could carve the words 'love', 'romance' or 'new boyfriend' or 'new girlfriend'. Put half a teaspoon of blessing seeds, also known as nigella seeds, into the mortar and grind to a powder with the pestle. Empty the powder onto a sheet of kitchen roll, anoint the candle in the oil then roll it through the blessing seed powder, pulling the candle towards you to draw love into your life as you say:

'A lover comes by candle's glow
From where or when I do not know
They come to me, true love to share
As the smokes curls through the air
As this wax melts, so do our hearts
Together a new life we start
And by the burning of this flame
Within three/two/one moons I will know their name
So mote it be.'

Melt the bottom of the candle and set it in the cauldron. Light the wick and allow it to burn down completely. Repeat with the next candle on the next full moon, adapting the final line of the incantation so that you are counting down the moons until your lover appears.

✦ Glamourie: Love Witch Spell

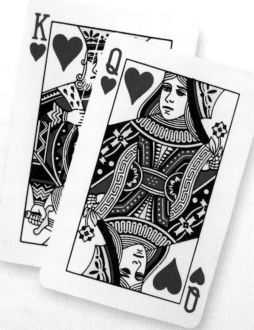

ITEMS REQUIRED: King or Queen of Hearts playing card, rose oil or rose water, a magnet.

TIMING: Perform on the new moon.

If you want to draw more love into your life, then use this spell to become a love magnet! On the night of the new moon, take the items to a quiet place where you will not be disturbed. Take the playing card and anoint the four corners, back and front, with rose oil or rose water, then gently brush the magnet across the image of the King or Queen, beginning at the crown and moving down towards the chest of the image. As you do so, chant the words:

> 'Like the King/Queen of Hearts,
> I am a magnet to love.'

Continue until you feel the magic *pop*, then place the playing card in your purse or wallet and carry it with you at all times. You should notice that you attract more romantic attention in the coming weeks and months.

Glamourie: White Rose Spell to Determine Someone's True Intentions

ITEMS REQUIRED: A single white rose, a white ribbon, a bud vase and water, a slip of paper and a red pen.

TIMING: Perform at the new moon.

Not everyone who flirts with you will have positive intentions. The white rose is a symbol of purity and it can be used to determine if your lover's intentions towards you are honourable or not. To begin with, write their name on the slip of paper in

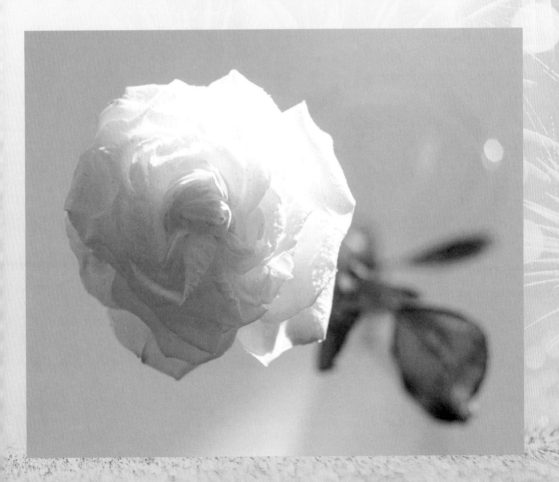

red ink. Use the ribbon to tie the name tag onto the stem of the rose. Hold your hands over the rose and say:

> 'A nagging doubt is in my mind so I must test their will
> Their true intentions I would find, be they good or ill
> Rose of love and purity, now tell all with your charm
> Is this lover true to me, or do they mean me harm?'

Place the rose in a bud vase of water and care for it well. If it blooms and opens wide, your lover's intentions towards you are pure and kind. If, however, the rose fails to open fully, then wilts and dies, they are holding secrets from you and their intentions are questionable. Let the rose be your guide.

Glamourie: Seed Spell to Choose Between Suitors

ITEMS REQUIRED: A pink, white or cream pillar candle, three (or however many suitors you have) pumpkin seeds, black felt-tip pen, lighter.

TIMING: Perform on the full to waning moon to whittle down the competition.

If you are a flower to bees (lucky you!) and you are having difficulty in choosing between suitors, then use this simple spell. First write the initial of each suitor onto one of the pumpkin seeds with the black pen. Next heat up the side of the candle with the lighter so that you can stick the seeds to the candle. Make sure that all the seeds are in a row, at the same height. Each suitor is now represented with a seed that bears his or her initial. Finally, light the wick of the candle. As the candle burns the seeds should fall, but the seed that lingers the longest represents the suitor you should choose, as they are the type to stick around.

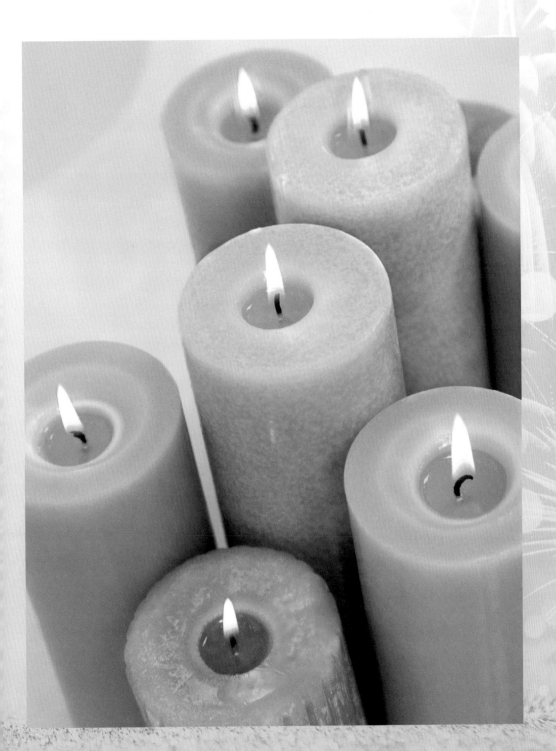

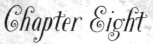

Chapter Eight

Lipstick, Powder and Paint

'I do not worry about my looks,
because beauty is not a
thing of age, but of spirit.'

VIVIEN LEIGH

People have used cosmetics and beauty treatments for centuries to enhance the way they look. From the powdered wigs, rouged cheeks and beauty marks of the 17th and 18th centuries, made famous by Marie Antoinette and Madame de Pompadour, to the vibrant New Romantics of the 1980s, both men and women alike have applied all kinds of makeup to transform their appearance.

Makeup could be thought of as real-life airbrushing – it conceals the flaws, makes eyes and lips appear larger, lashes longer and cheeks rosier. There is a certain kind of magic in makeup and it is the magic of illusion. It really is a smoke-and-mirrors trick, but far from being a frivolous feminine activity, makeup can be viewed as a magical tool in its own right. In this chapter we are going to explore the magic of makeup, beauty potions and how to cast spells using items that you might find on any dressing table.

BEAUTY IS ONLY SKIN DEEP

Loving the skin you are in is much easier if your skin feels like satin and smells divine. A good skincare routine is essential to keep your complexion clear and healthy. Different skin types need different kinds of care, but there are a couple of gentle home-made beauty products that suit most skin types. Ingredients can easily be found in the supermarket, or you might already have them in your kitchen cupboard. So, stir up some glamour magic with these simple home-made beauty treatments. Make sure to do a quick patch test of the remedy to ensure you have no allergic reactions. All these beauty potions should be used as soon as you have made them.

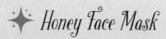

✦ *Glamourie:* ✦
MAKE YOUR OWN FACE MASKS

✦ *Honey Face Mask*

This one is good for all skin types, but is especially effective at soothing skin that is prone to spots and blemishes. All you need is about a tablespoon of pure honey and a brush to apply it with. Smear a layer of honey all over your face and neck. As you do so say:

> 'Mellona, Goddess of honey pure,
> Mask me in your gift of allure
> Clear my complexion, brighten my skin
> So that honey-dew glows from within.'

Leave the mask on for about 10-15 minutes, then gently wipe it off with a wash cloth. Tone and moisturize as usual.

✦ *Brightening Face Mask*

This mask is good for dull, tired skin. Natural yogurt is great for helping to remove dead skin cells, especially when mixed with a little turmeric. The yogurt will lift away the dead skin, while the turmeric will help to reduce hyper-pigmentation and redness.

Mix half a teaspoon of turmeric powder with a tablespoon of natural Greek yogurt. Make sure the ingredients are thoroughly mixed together, then apply all over face and neck, being careful to avoid the eye area, and say:

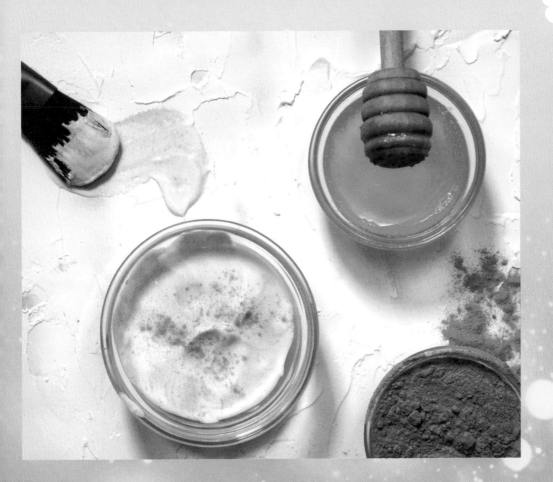

'Aphrodite, Greek goddess of love,
Brighten my charms with light from above.'

Leave the mask on for just 10 minutes – any longer and the turmeric can begin to irritate sensitive skin, then rinse it off, tone and moisturize.

✦ Tightening Face Mask

To reduce fine lines and tighten pores, separate the white from one large egg. Add a teaspoon of lemon juice to the egg white and whisk it together until it makes a foamy consistency, similar to meringue. Apply it all over your face and neck, saying:

> 'Cosmic eggs, refresh and renew
> Let my skin be as fresh as the morning dew.'

Leave for 10-15 minutes, then rinse off with cool water. Never use hot water on egg-based home-beauty products or the egg will begin to cook! This mask will leave your skin feeling quite taut as it minimizes the pores, so it is essential to moisturize well afterwards.

YOUR CROWNING GLORY

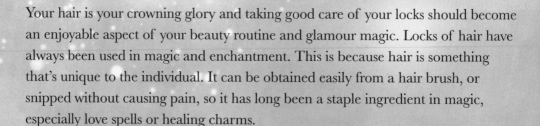

Your hair is your crowning glory and taking good care of your locks should become an enjoyable aspect of your beauty routine and glamour magic. Locks of hair have always been used in magic and enchantment. This is because hair is something that's unique to the individual. It can be obtained easily from a hair brush, or snipped without causing pain, so it has long been a staple ingredient in magic, especially love spells or healing charms.

Giving away a lock of your hair was a sign of complete trust, because it was said to give the receiver power over you. For this reason, in the past, a bride would often give a lock of her hair to the groom, to signify her obedience to his will and her trust in him. In modern magic, a popular love ritual involves tying together a lock of your hair with one from your partner using red thread and keeping this

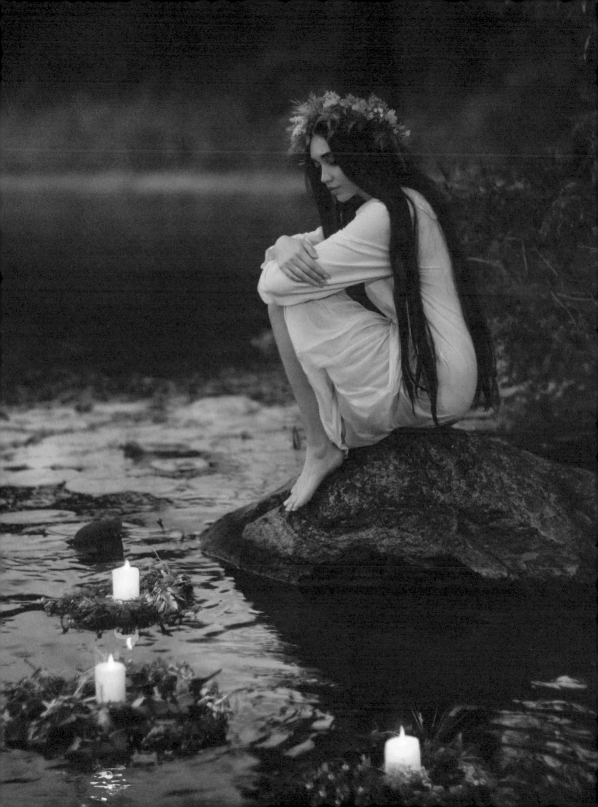

charm under the mattress. This would seal the bond between you and create a lasting love affair.

In terms of beauty magic, there are a few rituals believed to promote a healthy head of hair. While we might all have to face a bad hair day from time to time, adding a touch of whimsical magic to your haircare routine can't hurt. Here, then, are a few enchanting tips for glamorous hair:

- Rinse hair with pure spring water once a month to keep it soft and silky.
- Brush hair outdoors in sunlight or moonlight to make it shine and gleam.
- Cut hair during a waxing moon to encourage regrowth.
- If you suffer from migraines, trimming your hair on the first Friday of a new year is said to cure them for the coming year.
- Dropping your comb whilst untangling your hair with it is said to bring about a disappointment.
- Saying a brushing charm as you brush your hair is said to stimulate hair growth.
- If you spot that the moon is full while you are brushing your hair, then it's a good time to make a wish.
- Using rose water to mist your hair is said to bring admirers your way.

Glamourie: A Spell for Luscious Locks

ITEMS REQUIRED: A pair of scissors, a hairbrush, your preferred leave-in conditioner, hair oil treatment or hair fragrance mist.

For the best results this spell should be cast on a waxing moon; however, the brushing chant can be repeated daily if you wish. First cut a small lock of your hair and bury it in the earth, preferably beneath a willow tree. This will promote the growth and fullness of your hair. Next, brush the treatment oil through your hair as you chant the following brushing charm:

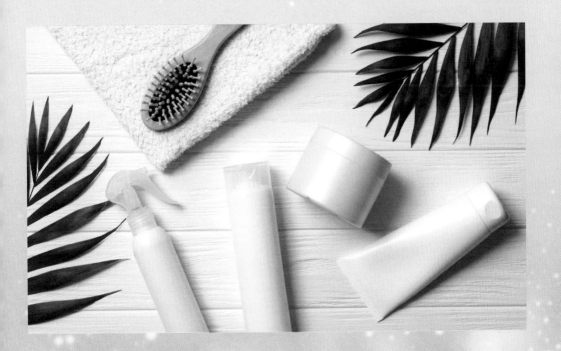

'Primp and preen and let it grow
Luscious locks, let them flow
Plait it, weave it, curl it round
In a ribbon tied and bound
Crimp it, wave it, pull it straight
Hanging lengths of swinging weight
Rumple, tousle and shake it well
To stir the growth of each follicle
From crown to waist in shining ream
I've the finest head of hair ever seen!'

THE EYES HAVE IT

Eyeliner is a staple product of many a beauty routine, but did you know that it was originally intended to be a form of magical protection? The Egyptians, who were famous for their elaborate eye makeup, wore eyeliner to ward off evil spirits and the 'evil eye' – that is, the spitefulness of others. It was also thought to protect the eyes from the harsh glare of the sun and to trap the dust of the desert before it got into the eyes. The Egyptians wore kohl all around their eyes, often in elaborate patterns. This was a way for them to show off their status and social standing, because the brightest pigments of green and blue came from semi-precious stones such as malachite and lapis lazuli. They would also use the juice of juniper berries to stain lips and cheeks.

The glamour of the Egyptians is undeniable and we can see how attached they were to their cosmetics, from the tombs, artefacts and grave goods that have been discovered over the years. Magic and makeup went hand in hand and people such as Cleopatra, Nefertiti and Tutankhamun would have been very intentional when they applied cosmetics, using makeup as a tool of magic and enchantment.

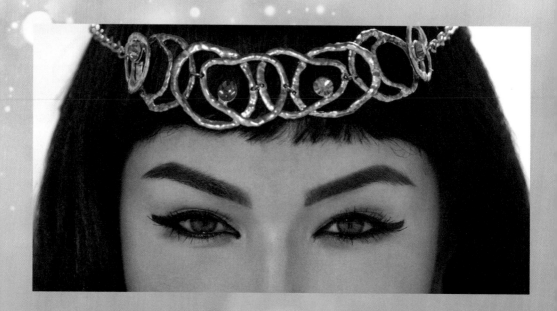

Glamourie: Cleopatra's Gaze Ritual

You can take a tip from the Egyptians by empowering your eyeliner and setting a magical intention as you apply it. First, hold the kohl pencil in your hands, close your eyes and empower it with these words:

'Eye of Horus, keep me calm
Guard me from all spite and harm
Lined in green and black and blue
Guard and guide me in all I do
Seeing clear, with eye of cat
Protected be from any mishap
So mote it be.'

Leave the eyeliner in the light of a full moon, then each time you use it, set the intention that you will see through anyone who presents a false face to you, or who would do you harm. According to Egyptian myth, the falcon-headed god Horus lost his left eye in a struggle with Seth, but the magical restoration of his eye came to symbolize the process of healing. With the eye of Horus on your side, you will be able quickly to avert any evil-eye energies that could be heading your way.

MAGIC DRIPS FROM SCARLET LIPS

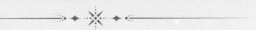

Red is the colour of success, victory and achievement. Wearing red can amplify the persona you have already created and make your spells more powerful. In magic, red is one of the power colours, along with black, and it is the best colour to wear if you want to be seen and turn heads. As the colour of blood, it is associated with the pagan mother goddess and the life force of sexual attraction. Red is also the colour attributed to a pagan priestess, so tap into your power as a witch by donning a scarlet-hooded coat, or a slick of red lipstick.

✦ *Glamourie: Make Your Own Lip Scrub*

ITEMS REQUIRED: One teaspoon of honey, two teaspoons of sugar, half a teaspoon of peppermint cordial.

Luscious lips should be soft and smooth, so give them some love with this pampering lip scrub. Mix all the ingredients together into a paste, then apply all over the lips in a circular motion to remove dead skin. Rinse off and apply lip balm to keep your lips in tiptop condition.

✦ *Glamourie: Siren's Kiss Lipstick Spell*

ITEMS REQUIRED: Lip balm, a red lipstick, a mint breath spray, a mirror.

Red lipstick is the epitome of glamour. From Hollywood royalty, such as Rita Hayworth to pop icon Taylor Swift, glamorous women have been wearing scarlet-red lips for decades. This little spell will ensure that you are heard by your target audience and that they will be hanging on your every word! It is a classic captivation

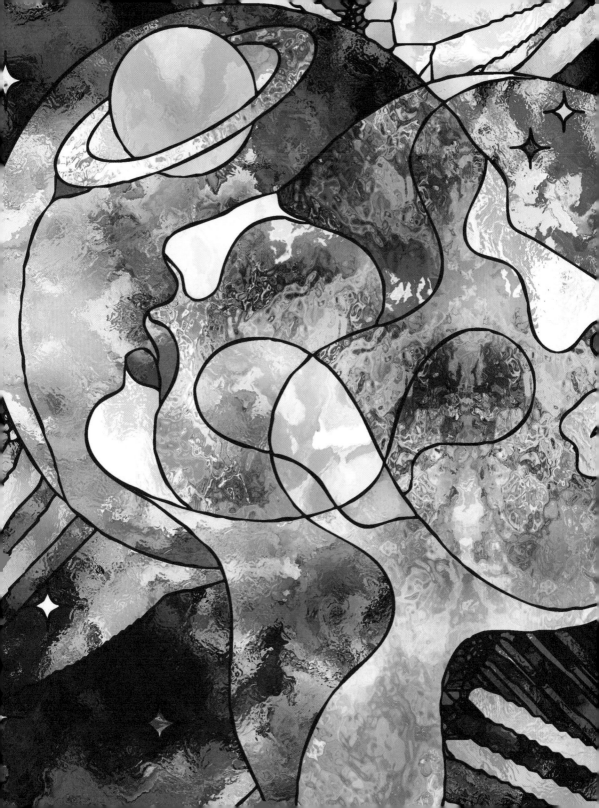

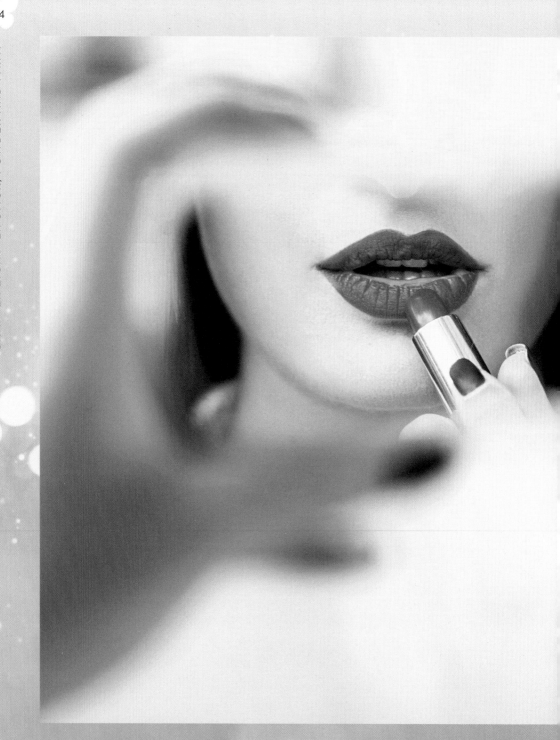

spell, designed to maximize your allure and draw people into your orbit. First, apply a lip balm to moisturize your lips. Next, use three pumps of the breath spray, visualizing your target audience being captivated by your voice. Mint is great for attraction spells and this step ensures that you will come across as being a 'breath of fresh air'. Finally, apply a perfect cupid's bow of red lipstick, look in the mirror and say:

'My voice is soft but my words hold power
I am captivating from this hour
A fascinating thread I weave
As my audience towards me cleaves
From scarlet lips sweet nothings fall
My red lips hold them all in thrall'

Be sure to keep the lipstick with you for any touch-ups to keep the magic strong.

✦ Glamourie: A Spell to Radiate Natural Beauty

ITEMS REQUIRED: A glass bowl, six tablespoons of witch hazel, six tablespoons of rose water, a sponge.

To maximize your allure and natural beauty, first pour the witch hazel and rose water into a bowl and stir. These are both natural ingredients, available in most chemists, and are often added to beauty products because they improve the complexion. Sit skyclad (naked) in front of a mirror and dip the sponge into the potion, then wipe it over your face and body, repeating this incantation three times:

'Aphrodite, hear my prayer
Your gift of beauty upon me share
Clear of skin and shining eyes
Inner beauty seldom lies
Here and now for all to see
I evoke my own unique beauty.'

Continue until you have used all the potion and repeat the ritual on each new moon to honour your inner beauty. After all, if you cannot honour and respect your own inner beauty, why expect anyone else to?

MIXOLOGY!

Never underestimate the power of mixology, which is when you mix pigments and fragrances together to create something completely new and unique to you. Try mixing two nail polishes or eyeshadows together to invent a whole new shade. Or perhaps layer a couple of perfumes, one on top of the other, to create a signature scent that no one else has. It goes without saying that this type of mixology should remain one of your beauty secrets, so don't tell anyone how you have achieved a look or scent that no one else can replicate, just let it be part of your alluring mystique!

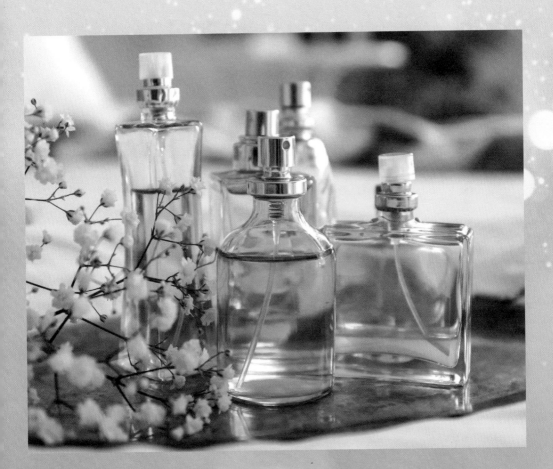

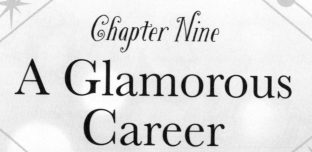

Chapter Nine

A Glamorous Career

'*I attribute my success to this – I never gave, or took an excuse.*'

FLORENCE NIGHTINGALE

Your career is a huge aspect of your life and it can be a leading cause of stress and mental health issues. If you dislike your job, it can be tough, but even a dream job will include tasks that you don't always enjoy. The days of a job 'for life' are long since over and suddenly finding yourself out of work, through no fault of your own, can be quite terrifying. In such circumstances, not only is it hard to remain optimistic, but with bills coming in and no salary to pay them, the future can look quite bleak. Furthermore, competition in the jobs market and workplace has never been fiercer, but with a few witch tricks up your sleeve, you can set yourself apart from the crowd and give yourself a magical edge.

Glamour might not be the first thing you think of when you imagine going in to work, but how you approach your work is entirely down to you. Even if you feel stuck in a job you hate, you can still make the most of your appearance and performance. Obviously your glam-o-meter should be turned to a low level when you are at work, but that doesn't mean that you should turn off the charm altogether. Remember that networking, socializing and team-building events are often when promotions are decided, so try to attend as many of these as you can and use some of the *glamouries* in this book to ensure that you look your best.

DRESS FOR THE JOB YOU WANT

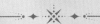

It might sound clichéd, but there is power in dressing for the job you want because it signals to the universe (and your boss!) that you are ready for the next step. Even if your dream job is nothing to do with your current employment, you can use your days off to dress for the career you *really* want. Invest in your dream by buying the kind of clothes you think you would wear in your ideal role, be that as a dancer, a writer, a beautician, or whatever your heart desires.

Your appearance counts for a lot when you are at work, so even if you have to wear a uniform, ensure that it is pressed properly, your shoes are polished and that you are well turned out at all times. Being organized is an asset too, so keep your desk tidy and your workload efficiently prioritized. This is a subtle way to add glamour to your work, because when you are organized and put together, you look as if you can handle greater responsibility. This is how promotions are subtly won.

AMBITION IS GLAMOROUS

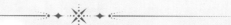

Glamorous people tend to be quite ambitious. They know what they want and they are not afraid to pursue their goals. Having ambition is a form of glamour in and of itself, because it indicates that you are not willing to settle for less than you deserve, or less than you are worth. Feeling undervalued at work can undermine your confidence and reduce job satisfaction. By contrast, developing your sense of ambition will give your confidence a boost because, even if you are currently in a dead-end job, your ambition will offer you a way out eventually. Letting people know that you have ambition will mean that you are more likely to be offered opportunities for extra training and so on, which, in turn, can help to further your ambition.

Bear in mind that attitude is everything, so even if the worst happens and you lose your job, it is vital that you remain optimistic and focused. Next time you visit the Jobcentre, take a look at the other people in the queue. Notice their body language and expressions. It's likely they'll be glum-faced with a slumped posture. Now do the exact opposite: stand tall, put your chin up and smile. Aim to look as if you could walk out of there and straight into any job of your choosing. Allow your ambition to show on your face, because you never know where your next opportunity is coming from and you need to look ready for it!

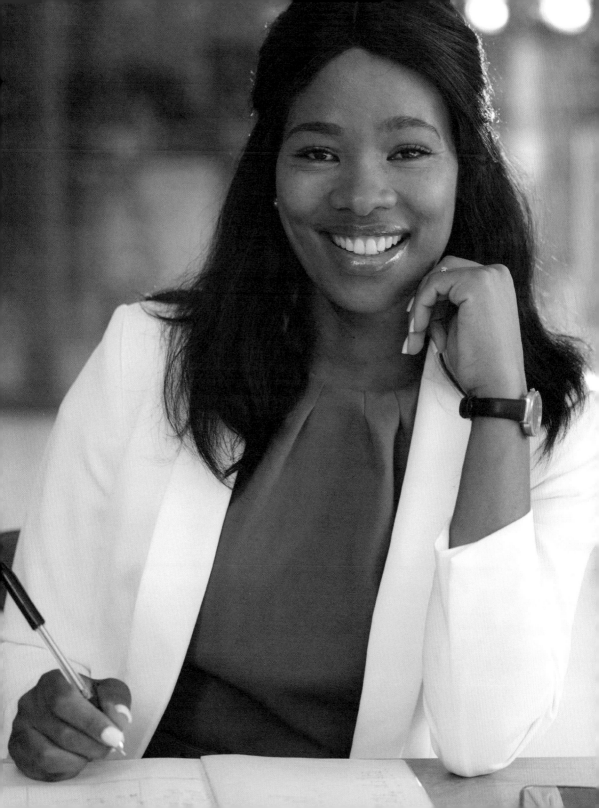

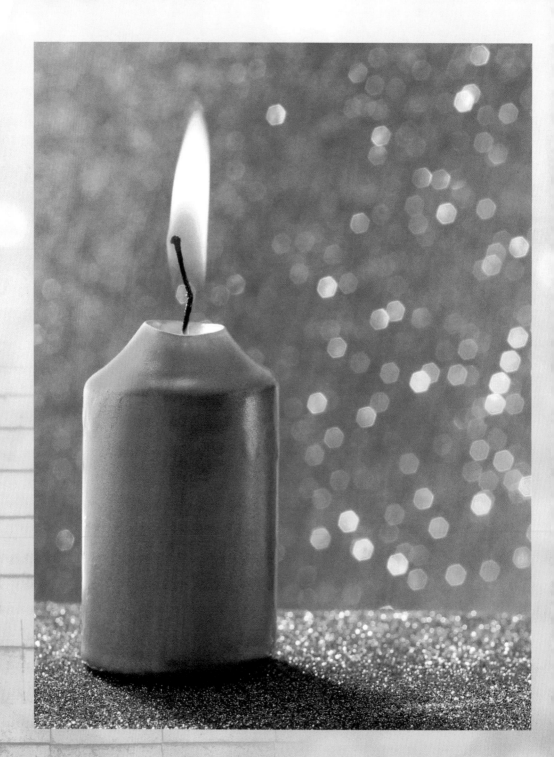

✦ Glamourie: Charm the Boss

ITEMS REQUIRED: A gold candle, a knife or carving tool, greaseproof paper.

If you have a job interview or you are interested in a promotion, you will want to make a good impression on the boss, so cast this simple spell. On a gold candle carve the name of the potential employer/promotion on one side and your own name on the other. Light the candle and chant this incantation for at least three minutes:

> 'A job within this fire be
> So hire/promote me, hire/promote me!
> A true employee I will be
> So hire/promote me, hire/promote me!'

Allow the candle to burn down naturally, but pour a little of the melted wax onto the greaseproof paper and let it set, then remove the wax and carry it with you to the interview to maintain a link with the magic you have made.

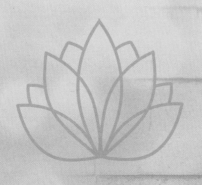

✦ Glamourie: Visualize Job Success

Interviews can be stressful and, when you're stressed, you rarely put in your best performance. You may not get every job you apply for, but you'll at least gain valuable interview experience. The more practised you are at interviews, the greater your chances of success, so when you find a job you really want, your nerves are less likely to let you down.

Remember that an interview works both ways. You should be taking the measure of the company just as much as they're sizing you up as an employee. So have a few questions prepared about the company as a whole and that branch of it in particular. For example, you might ask about their ethical practices, what steps they are taking to reduce their carbon footprint and so on. Once you have prepared

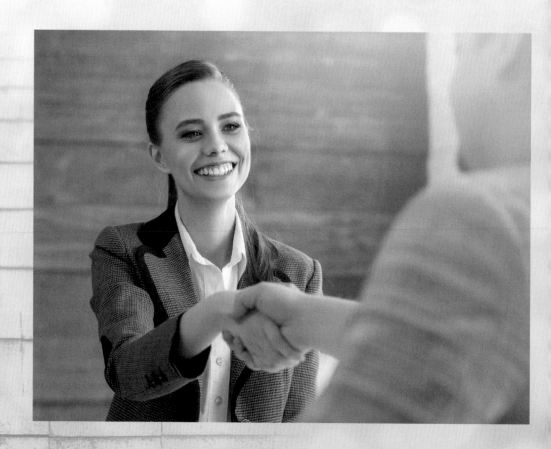

in this way, cast this spell the night before the interview to give yourself a magical advantage over the competition!

Hold a tealight between your palms and visualize yourself going through the interview process. See yourself as well-groomed, relaxed, giving clear and intelligent answers. Then light the tealight and say:

'In interviews I am the star
I outshine all the rest
This job/promotion is mine and well-deserved
For I pass every test!'

Leave the candle to burn down and spend the evening doing things that help to keep you feeling calm and relaxed, ready for the day ahead.

GLAMOROUS CAREERS

There is no doubt that some jobs are more glamorous than others, but all jobs are valid and vital to society. Where would we be without refuse collectors, couriers, receptionists or carers? There are some roles, however, that simply ooze glamour – think of fighter pilots, actors, models, ballet dancers, novelists and so on – while other roles seem much more mundane.

Although not everyone will be fortunate enough to make their career in a glamorous field of employment, we are all capable of bringing more glamour to the work that we do, with our personal appearance, presentation, attitude, ambition, organization and efficiency. Your working life will be as glamorous as you make it, so make it glimmer and gleam with magic!

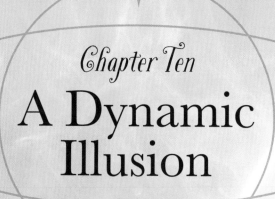

Chapter Ten
A Dynamic
Illusion

'Even I don't wake up
looking like Cindy Crawford!'

CINDY CRAWFORD

Glamour is a dynamic force. It isn't something that you achieve once and have forever, but it is something that you can spend your entire life cultivating and enjoying. Glamour is fluid: it changes as you change, with your perspective of glamour shifting as you age and move through different life stages. What felt glamorous to you in your youth, when you were focused on dating and finding a life partner, might not feel so important in later life. Ageing, parenting and your relationship status can all have an impact on what you perceive to be glamorous.

However, glamour is always there for the taking. It has no age limit and you can be just as glamorous at 70 as you were at 20, just in a different way. With longer life comes experience, knowledge, skills and competence, all of which can add to your overall glamour. As you age, you will become better at setting and maintaining personal boundaries and knowing your own worth. Nobody is so old that they can't exude an aura of glamour if they want to. It just means making that little bit of extra effort.

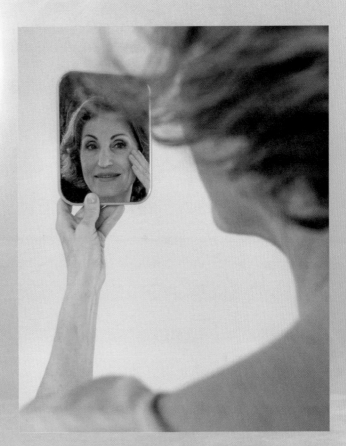

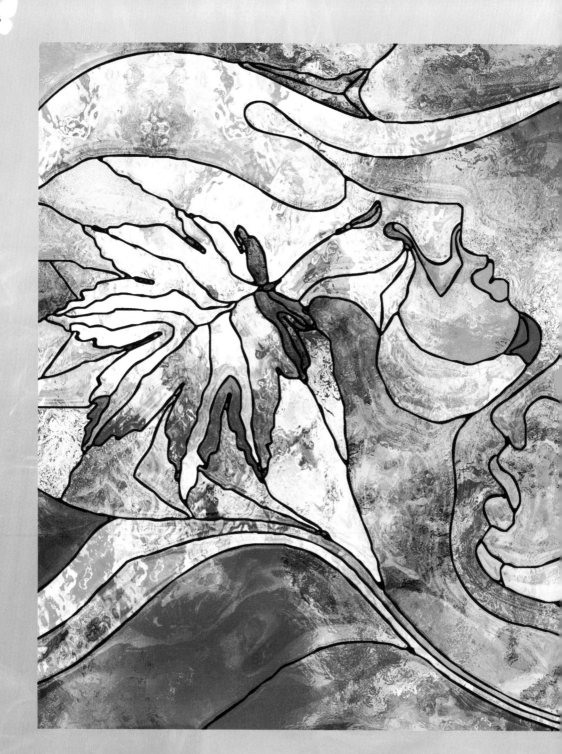

SHE'S LET HERSELF GO

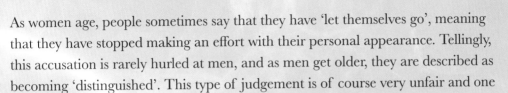

As women age, people sometimes say that they have 'let themselves go', meaning that they have stopped making an effort with their personal appearance. Tellingly, this accusation is rarely hurled at men, and as men get older, they are described as becoming 'distinguished'. This type of judgement is of course very unfair and one of many signs of the misogynistic double standards in our culture.

Ageing is a natural process and it happens to everyone who is lucky enough to live a long life. Try not to fear this process. Society will always set impossible beauty standards, but you can, and should, continue to set your own, regardless of how old you are. But you should do this for you and your relationship with yourself, which are more important than any external judgement coming from a patriarchal culture.

DOWN DAYS AND DARK NIGHTS OF THE SOUL

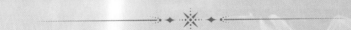

There will be times over the course of your life when troubles weigh you down and your mental health suffers. Illness, bereavement, family dramas and relationship woes can all have an impact on how you feel about yourself. There will also be days when you simply can't be bothered to look glamorous! That's fine. Everyone is allowed a few off-days every now and then and glamour should never feel like a chore on your to-do list. It should feel like self-care, for that is what it is. As we said at the start of the book, looking good can help you to *feel* better, so rather than forgoing your glamour altogether during the difficult seasons of your life, think ahead and prepare for those times instead.

✦ Glamourie: Create a Glamour Chest

A glamour chest is something you can turn to when you are feeling down, when you have low energy and you're not up to leaving the house. It doesn't have to be a chest. It could be a drawer, a cupboard or a box tucked into the bottom of the wardrobe or under the bed. The idea of it is that you have a stash of treats available to you when you need them. Once you have decided where your glamour chest is going to be, set about filling it with all the little treats you know will help to make you feel better. Here are a few hints of items for your chest to get you started:

- A couple of biodegradable sheet face masks. These are easily used and then thrown away, leaving less mess to clean up afterwards.
- A foot mask and a luxurious foot cream.
- Bath bombs or shower steamers to make bathing more luxurious.

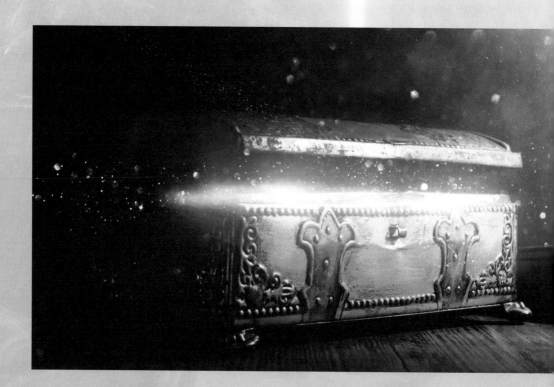

- Lavender essential oil or a lavender pillow spray. These will add a healing scent to your sheets and pillows if you are stuck in bed fighting off a chest infection.
- Lip balm and hand cream, because small acts of pampering are good for you, and these take no energy to apply.
- An exciting new novel that you have never read before.
- A favourite childhood book to re-read for the nostalgia.
- A book of poems.
- An uplifting playlist, and also one of softer music that you can fall asleep to.
- A box of special tea that you only use when you are feeling under the weather. Gingerbread, blackcurrant, mulled wine and sleepy teas are all good ones to try.
- A sweet-smelling hand sanitizer to keep any germs under control.
- A pair of fluffy bed socks and a hot water bottle to cuddle.
- Luxury hot chocolate.
- A scented candle to cast a warm glow.
- A tin of peppermint sweets or lozenges.

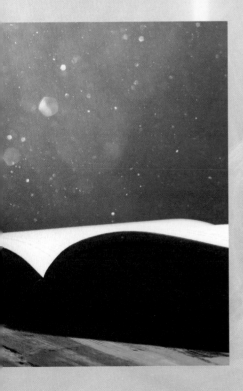

Prepare your glamour chest so it is as comforting and well-stocked as possible. When the worst happens and life takes a dark and unexpected turn, you will already have everything you need to pamper yourself. Treat yourself like a favoured child throughout any dark nights of the soul and allow your glamour to shine more gently.

✦ Glamourie: A Restorative Lavender Bath Potion

ITEMS REQUIRED: A voile pouch, muslin cloth or hankie, two teaspoons of dried lavender, one teaspoon of dried camomile flowers, a lavender ribbon, lavender essential oil.

If there is a more restful way to destress than soaking in a fragrant lavender bath, I haven't found it yet. This is one of my staple remedies. For this restorative bath potion, you will need two parts dried lavender, mixed with one part dried camomile flowers. Both these herbs are well known for their healing and restful properties. First make the bathroom enticing. Light candles if you want to and run a hot bath. Place the dried herbs into the pouch, or in the middle of the hankie and tie it tightly using the ribbon.

As the bath fills, swirl the pouch of herbs in the water in a clockwise direction, scenting the hot water with fragrance. Imagine that once you sink into the water, all your cares will float away on lavender clouds. Tie the pouch to the tap so that it hangs in the water. As a final step, add 10 drops of lavender essential oil to the water just before you sink into the depths. Relax and breathe in the fragrance. Allow the herbal scent to calm you and let go of any stressful thoughts.

Remain in the water for as long as you can, making the most of the restful energies of the herbs. When you are ready, dry off and empty the wet herbs into the earth, giving back what you have taken. Enjoy the remainder of your day and do calming, gentle activities to maintain your sense of peace. You can also use this pouch in a shower, hanging it by the shower head and letting the steam release the scents.

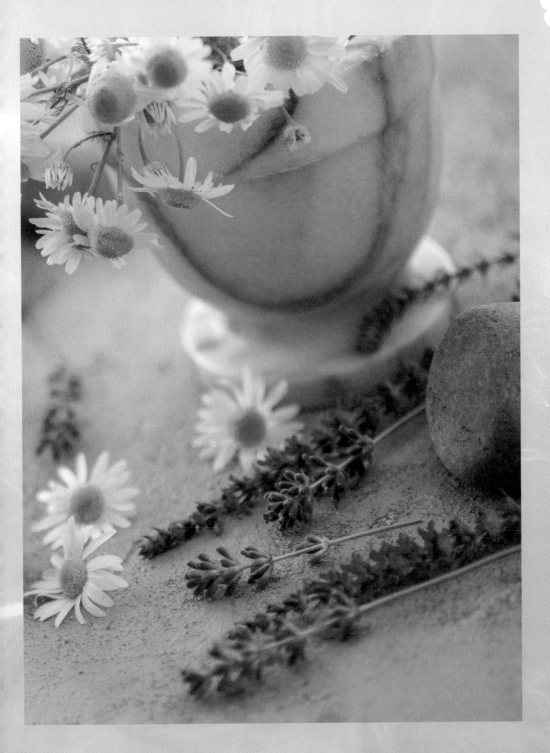

Conclusion

Glamour Is Soul Craft

'*I feel glamorous on the inside,
so I want to look like it on the outside.*'

DOLLY PARTON

I hope that you have found this little book of glamour spells interesting and enticing. Glamour is a form of soul craft, for it can lift the spirits and calm the chatter of the mind. Hopefully, making time for pampering yourself will become a priority for you, while adding a touch of magic means that your life is, in turn, touched by all the enchantment of *glamourie*! People will perceive you differently and they will begin to ask what your secret is. You are likely to receive more attention, more compliments, kind gifts and favours. All this is down to the glamour that you have cast around yourself.

You are the star of your own life, so step out into the world dazzling and delighting everyone you meet. Your aura is glimmering, your spirit is strong, your natural beauty glows. Put your best face forward and go and make your dreams come true. After all, that's what *glamouries* are all about – making your beautiful dreams a reality. Embrace the illusion until it becomes real and know that you have the power to captivate an audience and charm people, wherever you go. May *glamourie* be always upon you and your life.

Beautiful blessings,

Marie Bruce x

FURTHER READING

✦ By the same author

Wicca
Celtic Spells
Moon Magic book and card deck
Book of Spells
Green Witchcraft
Wicca for Self-Transformation
Moon Magic
Celtic Magic book and card deck

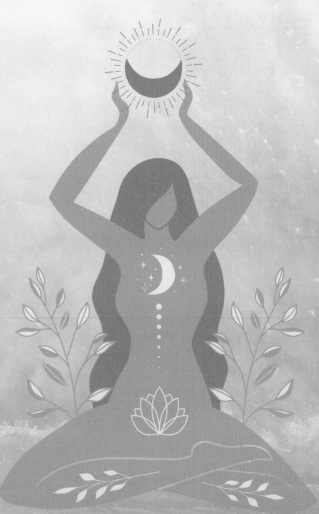

✦ *Books on glamour*

BRUCE, Marie (2008). *The Wiccan Temptress*. London, Hale Books

CASTELLANO, Deborah (2021). *Glamour Magic*. USA, Llewellyn Publications

DOWNING, Sarah Jane (2018). *Beauty and Cosmetics 1550–1950*. Oxford, Shire Publications

DUBBERLEY, Emily (2005). *Things a Woman Should Know About Seduction*. London, Carlton Publishing

GOYDER, Caroline (2009). *The Star Qualities*. London, Pan Macmillan

HOMER, Karen (2005). *Things a Woman Should Know About Beauty*. London, Carlton Publishing

HOMER, Karen (2003). *Things a Woman Should Know About Style*. London, Carlton Publishing

HUNTER, Adriana (1994). *Etiquette: A Guide to Modern Manners*. Glasgow, HarperCollins

YOUNG, Louise with SHEPPARD, Loulia (2017). *Timeless: A Century of Iconic Looks*. London, Octopus Publishing

VON TEESE, Dita with APODACA, Rose (2015). *Your Beauty Mark: The Ultimate Guide to Eccentric Glamour*. New York, HarperCollins

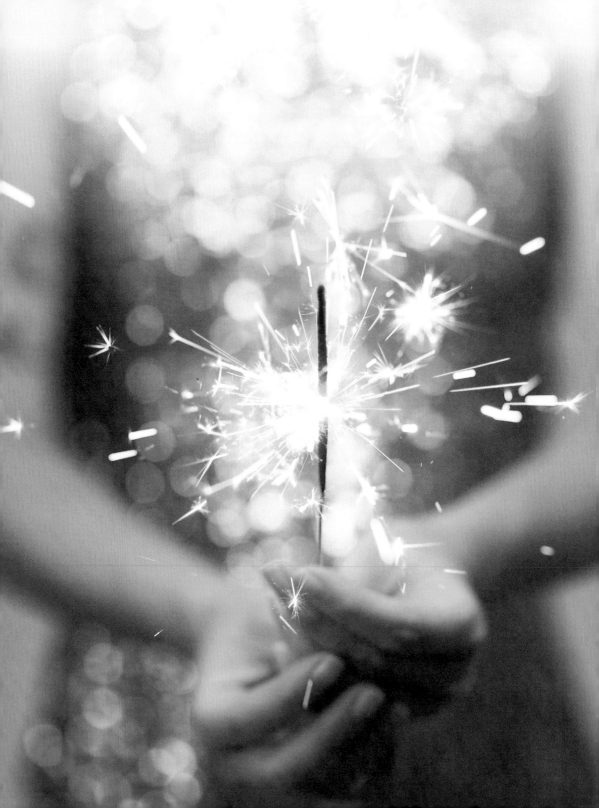

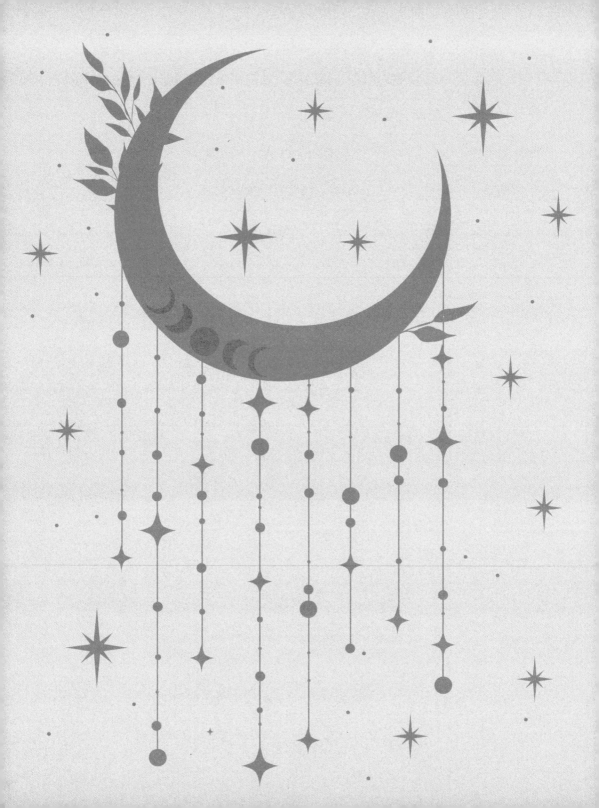